P9-BIT-916

Neural Network Principles

ROBERT L. HARVEY, Ph.D.

Lincoln Laboratory
Massachusetts Institute of Technology

PRENTICE HALL, Englewood Cliffs, New Jersey 07632

Library of Congress Cataloging-in-Publication Data

Harvey, Robert L.
    Neural network principles / Robert L. Harvey.
        p.   cm.
    Includes bibliographical references and index.
    ISBN 0-13-063330-5
    1. Neural networks (Neurobiology)   I. Title.
    [DNLM: 1. Nerve Net.   2. Models, Neurological.   WL 102 H342n
    1994]
    QP363.3.H37   1994
    612.8–dc20   93-42660
                                                                CIP

Acquisitions editor: DON FOWLEY
Project manager: JENNIFER WENZEL
Copy editor: MARTHA WILLIAMS
Cover designer: RAY LUNDGREN GRAPHICS, LTD.
Buyer: DAVE DICKEY
Editorial assistant: JENNIFER KLEIN

©1994 by Prentice-Hall, Inc.
A Paramount Communications Company
Englewood Cliffs, New Jersey 07632

The author and publisher of this book have used their best efforts in preparing this book. These efforts include the development, research, and testing of the theories and programs to determine their effectiveness. The author and publisher make no warranty of any kind, expressed or implied, with regard to these programs or the documentation contained in this book. The author and publisher shall not be liable in any event for incidental or consequential damages in connection with, or arising out of, the furnishing, performance, or use of these programs.

Note: Figure credits appear on pages 186–87.

Printed in the United States of America

10 9 8 7 6 5 4 3 2 1

> *With love and affection*
> *for Rosie,*
> *Cara, Alyson, and Max*

ISBN 0-13-063330-5

Prentice-Hall International (UK) Limited, *London*
Prentice-Hall of Australia Pty. Limited, *Sydney*
Prentice-Hall Canada, Inc., *Toronto*
Prentice-Hall Hispanoamericana, S.A., *Mexico*
Prentice-Hall of India Private Limited, *New Delhi*
Prentice-Hall of Japan, Inc., *Tokyo*
Simon & Schuster Asia Pte. Ltd., *Singapore*
Editora Prentice-Hall do Brasil, Ltda., *Rio de Janeiro*

Contents

Preface

Neural networks is a subject lying at the intersection of psychology, mathematics, neuro-science, and systems theory. Currently this field is experiencing rapid development because of its applications. The applications include robotics, pattern recognition (for speech and vision systems), and understanding human brain-mind processes. This volume presents the basic ideas of neural networks.

The point of view is modeling biological nervous systems. This powerful and elegant approach to neural networks is attractive because it pushes system design toward the higher-performing biological systems. Moreover, these biological models give a springboard for a broad range of applications.

The text develops neural network theory and design principles as follows.

Chapters 1 and 2 outline the structure of the human brain, the physics of neurons, and derive the standard neuron state equations. In a sense, the remainder of the book presents the consequences of solving these equations.

Chapter 3 derives a set of simple networks. These networks can filter, recall, switch, amplify, and recognize input signals (patterns of neuron activation). Neural networks can also account for many experimental psychology results.

Chapter 4 discusses properties of general neuron groups. Adaptive resonance theory neural networks (ART-1 and ART-2) combine several functions simultaneously and can serve as memory modules. The chapter discusses the well-known Hopfield and perceptron neural networks by this unified biological approach, including new design procedures for both.

Chapters 5 and 6 apply the theory to synthesize neural networks for specialized tasks. These systems can process data from a variety of sensors and can approach human performance.

Chapter 5 outlines the design of machine vision systems. The chapter describes an architecture for a general purpose system that can learn to recognize stationary objects—such as vehicles or cancer cells—in their natural background.

Chapter 6 outlines motor control in human beings. It then presents two examples of robotic hand-eye systems.

Chapter 7 turns to the mathematical task of solving large systems of interconnected neurons. A very simple genetic algorithm gives new techniques for designing complex neural networks with fixed arbitrary connections. These modules can function as preprocessors, controllers, and feature detectors in complex systems.

Chapter 8 outlines global control and modulation in the human brain-mind. This material leads to a new understanding of many mental illnesses. Indeed, explaining human mental functions is an emerging application of neural networks.

Chapter 9 ends this volume by briefly considering some philosophical issues—especially consciousness—from a neural network view. Though perhaps controversial, these issues are nevertheless at the heart of many students' and researchers' interest in neural networks. In a sense, this short chapter may point to the next major milestone—designing neural networks that mimic high-level human processes.

The course for which this text is designed normally carries a prerequisite of courses in conventional signal processing. An effort was made, however, to keep the book self-contained.

The mathematical background needed is the customary undergraduate courses in advanced calculus, linear algebra, and ordinary differential equations. An elementary acquaintance with control theory and its simpler concepts of stability, is helpful for understanding general cooperative-competitive systems.

The exercises of each chapter have been limited to those extending the text, or illustrating a point. Pedantic museum pieces have been avoided. A solutions manual is available for instructors from the publisher. Some exercises may provoke original thought; some could be developed in a thesis.

References at the end of each chapter amplify the material discussed or treat points not touched on. The accompanying evaluations are purely personal, of course. It was felt necessary, however, to provide the student with some guide to the bewildering maze of literature on neural networks. The bibliography at the end of the book lists these references, along with many more. The list is not intended to be complete in any sense. The list contains the references used in writing this book. Thus, it serves to acknowledge my debt to these sources.

Notation is always a vexing question. Achieving a consistent, practical, unambiguous system of notation is impossible. A separate index at the end of the book lists the initial appearance of important symbols. Minor characters, appearing only once, are not included.

Terminology is also a bothersome issue, especially so with a subject cutting across many highly developed fields. To mitigate terminology problems, a glossary at the end of the book has common terms from philosophy, psychology, neuroscience, and neuroanatomy.

The present text evolved from courses on neural networks I taught at Northeastern University during 1990 to 1992 in the Graduate School of Engineering and the State-of-the-Art program. I am grateful to Professor John Proakis, chairman of the Northeastern

University Department of Electrical and Computer Engineering, for many personal and official encouragements. I also wish to record my deep gratitude to the students in my courses. Their favorable reactions provided the impetus for this work.

I would like to thank Doctor Peter G. Anderson of the Rochester Institute of Technology, Doctor John Wu of Auburn University, and Professor N. K. Bose, HRB Systems Professor and Director of the Spatial and Temporal Signal Processing Center of the Pennsylvania State University, for reviewing the manuscript and offering valuable suggestions. The responsibility of the present book rests with me, of course. Suggestions are welcome.

I wish to thank M.I.T. Lincoln Laboratory for providing support and for a stimulating environment in which the book could be developed.

Finally, I wish to acknowledge others who helped me during this project: Gail Carpenter, Mike Carter, Paul DiCaprio, Dan Dudgeon, John Dugan, Mary Fouser, Stephen Grossberg, Alfred Gschwendtner, Karl Heinemann, David Hestenes, Patrick Hirschler-Marchand, Eric Kandel, Ernest Kent, Gloria Liias, Courosh Mehanian, Murali Menon, Charles Niessen, Linda Peterson, Barney Reiffen, Mark Silverman, Alex Sonnenschein, John Uhran, and Rose Harvey.

Robert L. Harvey

1

Introduction

Intelligent machines with huge numbers of simple elements was a research subject for many science pioneers. References to this subject can be found in the scientific literature of the nineteenth century and, with increasing frequency, into the 1950s. Starting in the late fifties, a field known as neural networks (NNs) evolved. Today NNs is distinct from signal processing, artificial intelligence (AI), and neuroscience, though it overlaps these fields and others.

The purpose of this book is to develop NN principles from a biological viewpoint, to give NN design methods for applications, and to outline human brain-mind functioning by a NN model.

Any scientific brain-mind theory has a number of fundamental concepts, such as memory and consciousness. The notion of these and other concepts will be examined briefly. For the most part, however, many fundamental concepts will be assumed as terms whose meanings are familiar. A glossary summarizes some terms from contributing disciplines.

1.1 ROAD MAP FOR NEURAL NETWORKS

NNs is part of systems theory because of its mathematical style [6,18]. Figure 1.1 is a simplified road map of current systems theory. The selected topics are familiar to students in many fields, especially engineering. As shown, the figure defines the branches of systems theory by their main characteristics.

To the left in figure 1.1 are topics in conventional signal processing. These subjects are the basic tools for designing modern electronic systems. Typically, the first years of an electrical engineering or a computer engineering graduate program introduce these subjects.

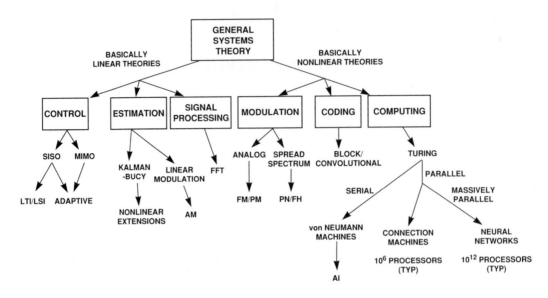

Figure 1.1   A simplified road map of systems theory. The major branches and subjects are shown. Neural networks is along a nonlinear branch. All branches share terminology, mathematical techniques, and with interpretation, results. Physics, chemistry, and the life sciences also contribute to neural networks and to the other branches.

To the right in figure 1.1 are branches of computing theory. AI is shown as being primarily serial processing, though much AI research is independent of the computer technology. For simplicity figure 1.1 omits many subdivisions of AI.

NNs branches from parallel processing on a branch labeled "massively parallel processing" by, say, one billion and more elements. The number of elements distinguishes NNs from connection machines. The NN branch, however, refers to the theory, not implementation, because current NNs rarely have more than a few thousand elements.

Figure 1.2 is the first of many definitions. The figure shows a NN schematically.

A <u>neural network</u> is a dynamical system with one-way interconnections. It carries out processing by its response to inputs. The processing elements are the nodes; the interconnects are directed links. Each processing element has a single output signal from which copies fan out.

Researchers approach NNs from many disciplines. Summarizing all the current approaches is difficult, because NNs is in rapid transition. Nevertheless, from an architectural viewpoint, current NN theory has three main branches: perceptron, associative memory, and biological model. These are suggestive labels, not standard terminology. Figure 1.3 shows the three branches and some leading researchers associated with each branch.

The perceptron branch, associated with Rosenblatt, is the oldest (late 1950s) and most developed. Currently, most NNs are perceptrons of one form or another (see section 4.4).

The associative memory branch is the source of the current revival in NNs (see section 4.3). Many researchers trace this revival to John Hopfield's 1982 paper (see chapter 1 references).

of the 52 Brodmann maps. Relating Brodmann area to function is often straightforward, for example, areas 17, 18, and 19 are associated with vision. Recent studies suggest the neocortex has at most about 200 modules and that finer subdivision is probably not helpful for understanding its operation.

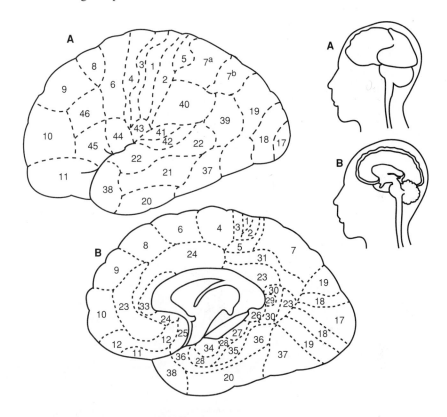

Figure 1.5 Brodmann's map of the human brain. The numbered areas chiefly reflect cell structure. Some are also connected to function. For example, areas 17, 18, and 19 are associated with vision. (From The Diagram Group. *The Brain—A User's Manual.* Reprinted by permission of Diagram Visual Information Limited, 1987; originally from Brodmann, 1908.)

Besides the anatomical description is the system description. Table 1.2 summarizes the major brain-mind systems and their functions. As shown, the major brain systems are sensory, motor, internal regulation, behavioral, and emotional. Research shows that each system is distributed over many areas of the brain.

To operate, the brain needs I/O signals. Major I/O channels to the outside world are the 12 pairs of cranial nerves, shown in figure 1.6 and described in table 1.3. As shown, some nerve bundles are one-way; others are two-way.

Other I/O channels are along the spinal cord (in an evolutionary sense the brain is an outgrowth of the spinal cord). The spine gets sensor signals, sends commands to the muscles, and makes simple decisions (reflex actions).

TABLE 1.2 MAJOR BRAIN SYSTEMS AND
THEIR FUNCTIONS

System	Function
Sensory	Vision
	Hearing
	Olfaction
	Taste
	Somatic sensation
Motor	Reflexes
	Movement of joints
Internal regulation	Appetite
	Sex
	Salt/water balances
Behavioral	Sleeping/waking
	Attention
Limbic	Emotions
	(motivation and priorities)

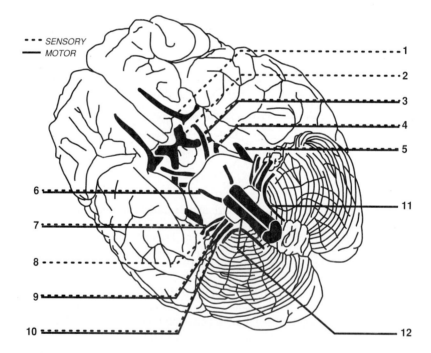

Figure 1.6 Schematic diagram of the cranial nervous system. Twelve pairs
of nerves are important input-output signal paths to the brain. Table 1.3 describes their function. (From The Diagram Group. *The Brain—A User's Manual.*
Reprinted by permission of Diagram Visual Information Limited, 1987.)

TABLE 1.3   THE CRANIAL NERVES AND THEIR FUNCTION

Nerve (12 Pairs)	Signal Direction	Sense	Motor
1. Olfactory	I	Smell	—
2. Optic	I	Vision	—
3. Oculomotor	I and O	—	Eye motion
4. Trochlear	I and O	—	Eye motion
5. Trigeminal	I and O	Facial sensations	Jaw motion
6. Abducens	I and O	Facial sensations	Eye motion
7. Facial	I and O	Taste	Facial expressions
8. Acoustic	I	Hearing	—
9. Glossopharyngeal	I and O	Taste	Pharynx/speech
10. Vagus	I and O	Breathing/heartbeat/digestion	
11. Accessory	O	—	Neck/shoulders
12. Hypoglossal	O	—	Tongue/speech

I = input to brain; O = output from brain.

As shown in table 1.4, at intervals along the spine, 31 nerve pairs pass through gaps in the surrounding bone vertebras.

TABLE 1.4   THE SPINAL NERVES AND FUNCTIONS

Spinal group	Nerve pairs	Body area
Cervical	8	Throat, chest, arms, hands
Thoracic	12	Top of breast bone to bottom of ribs
Lumbar	5	Front of legs and feet
Sacral	5	Soles of feet and back of legs
Coccygeal	1	Soles of feet and back of legs

Several million cranial nerves link the brain to sense organs in the head, and about 10 million nerves run from the brain to the spinal cord.

The five traditional senses are sight, hearing, smell, taste, and touch. For reference, table 1.5 summarizes some characteristics of human vision, hearing, and touch [82].

The minimum perceptible visual input approaches the quantum mechanical limit for detecting photons (see chapter 1 exercises). Human vision also has, in engineering terminology, a dynamic range of 90 dB and a relative color discrimination of 7 bits.

Standard terminology for I/O is as follows. Nerve endings are one of three kinds. Exteroceptors bring information from outside the body, for example, vision. Interoceptors bring information originating from within the body. Proprioceptors bring information about joint position and muscle tension. The direction of signal flow is either afferent (input) or efferent (output).

Standard terminology for naming brain regions is as follows. Some brain structures are superior (above) or inferior (below). Names of brain structures are also from the bone

TABLE 1.5 SELECTED CHARACTERISTICS OF THREE PRIMARY HUMAN SENSES (From Sheridan and Ferrel. *Man-Machine Systems.* Adapted by permission of the MIT Press, 1974)

Attribute	Vision	Hearing	Touch
Minimum perceptible magnitude	3×10^{-10}erg	10^{-9}erg/cm^2	3×10^{-2} erg
Maximum tolerable magnitude	10^9 times min	10^{13} times min	10^2 times minimum
Relative magnitude discrimination	570	325 at midfreq	15 at 200–300 Hz
Absolute magnitude discrimination	5–7 steps on gray scale	5–7 steps at 1000 to 2000 Hz	5–7 steps at 200 to 300 Hz
Frequency range	0.3 to 1.5 μm	20 to 20,000 Hz	0 to 10,000 Hz
Relative frequency discrimination	128	1800 at 60 dB	200
Absolute frequency discrimination	12–13 hues	5–9 up to 80 for perfect pitch	depends on skin area

covering the structure. Thus, the inferior temporal cortex (ITC) is the brain area below and under the temporal bone (area 20 in figure 1.5).

Considering gross mental functioning, evidence from brain-damaged individuals suggests the cortex halves have specialized functions. Localizing function in brain areas is an active research topic, and research is refining the findings.

To a first approximation, for most individuals, the right hemisphere processes information as complete patterns and is sensitive to, for example, static shapes.

The left hemisphere processes information sequentially (or dynamically), and thus is involved in, for example, speech and language. The vision areas lie in the two hemispheres and thus are sensitive to pattern and motion.

In human brain functioning, research has two major directions: localizing function and discovering mechanisms. Localization usually tells little about the logical operations of brain function. Localization, however, can sometimes set limits on the processing (see chapter 1 exercises).

Discovery of mechanisms is limited by experimental techniques, especially for complex behavior. The limitations include recording time of a neuron, methods for recording from millions of neurons, and the means for storing and interrelating data. Many researchers believe a computer simulation might be the best explanation for various kinds of behavior.

Research shows neuron structure and signaling are remarkably similar throughout the brain. That is, meaning is associated with brain area and not the kind of signal. Thus, "seeing" is signals in the vision system; "hearing" is signals in the auditory system.

The phenomenon of consciousness interests students and researchers alike. Consciousness is a difficult phenomenon to define, let alone model or build into machines. Indeed, many researchers distinguish between consciousness and self-awareness.

Consciousness, many believe, resides in the reticular formation, a group of cells within the brain stem. Nerves from this area go to all parts of the midbrain and forebrain and arouse these regions. The reticular formation is likened to a power supply driving the neocortex.

Without reticular signals the brain grows sleepy. Damage to the reticular formation causes unconsciousness; irreversible reticular damage causes coma.

Self-awareness is the result of neocortex activity, according to many theories. Edelman's theory (1977) [29] postulates that awareness is interchanging signals among neuron groups. In Edelman's theory, matching current inputs and stored memories produces what we call awareness. Nonawareness corresponds to nonmatching between these patterns.

Self-awareness is explained by Dennett (1991) [26] as many simultaneous, parallel brain activities. Indeed, the phenomenon cannot be localized in time or area. Dennett's model also explains many findings and paradoxes.

Recently a wholly biological mechanism for self-awareness is emerging from physical findings, summarized by Black [8] (see chapter 2). Self-awareness is taken up again in chapter 9 and discussed briefly by the NN theory developed in the intervening text.

In summary, the basic hypothesis of this book is that brain-mind functioning, normal and abnormal, is explainable by its structure. These functions include moving, sensing, and talking. The hypothesis also includes "higher functions" such as hoping, dreaming, and thinking.

This hypothesis, however, is controversial and some writers have challenged a wholly physical model for the human brain-mind system (see chapter 1 references).

The traditional paradigm of philosophy and cognition science is that an objective reality "out there" is simply mirrored by mental representations "in here." Moreover, the categories of individuals for classifying experiences are universal and invariant.

The new paradigm, suggested by NN theory and the life sciences, is that mental processes emerge from physical mechanisms. Indeed, the classifying categories are from prototypes defined in unique and unexpected ways. Chapter 9 considers some philosophical implications.

SUGGESTED REFERENCES[1]

F. Bloom, *Brain, Mind, and Behavior* and The Diagram Group, *The Brain—A User's Manual*. These are two surveys of neuroscience for the educated reader. They have many well-drawn sketches and diagrams. Bloom's book was written as part of a teaching package for a TV series and has a psychological viewpoint, while the Diagram Group has a medical viewpoint. Both are nonmathematical.

S. Goldberg, *Clinical Neuroanatomy made Ridiculously Easy*. This is a book intended to help nurses, medical students, and paramedical personnel master essential parts of neuroanatomy. The book is brief and readable. It gives many examples of dysfunctions. The mnemonics and humor in this book are an effective educational device, which unfortunately is not frequently tried in academic education.

E. Kent, *The Brains of Men and Machines*. An excellent book describing human brain architecture by processing modules. Although it does not treat neural networks, it has descriptions of perceptual functions, for example vision, written from a signal processing point of view. The book is nonmathematical with many block diagrams.

---

[1] For convenience the references at the end of each chapter are listed only by short title. Full bibliographical description will be found in the bibliography at the end of the book.

R. PENROSE, *The Emperor's New Mind*. This book discusses computers, minds, and the laws of physics on an advanced level. Penrose argues for a non-algorithmic basis for consciousness. The book challenges the basic hypothesis of the text. This book can serve as an excellent point of departure for reading on the basic ideas involved in neural networks. The mathematics is at a senior undergraduate level.

D. RUMELHART, *Parallel Distributed Processing*. This two-volume book is a standard reference and is a unique source for many specialized topics. Chapter 20 is an excellent summary of anatomy and physiology of the cerebral cortex.

G. EDELMAN and V. MOUNTCASTLE, *The Mindful Brain*. The first chapter describes Mountcastle's column organization of the cerebral cortex, a major finding in neuroscience. The second chapter by Edelman connects the column structure of neuron groups (originated by Mountcastle) to consciousness. A theory of consciousness is an active research area, and new results are published monthly. These two chapters are excellent background to current research.

M. MINSKY and S. PAPERT, *Perceptrons: An Introduction to Computational Geometry*. Many researchers credit this classical and controversial (1960s) book with stopping research in highly parallel networks (a claim denied by the authors). Hopfield's paper later revived interest in neural networks. Minsky and Papert based their arguments on two-layer perceptrons (see chapter 4). Most of Minsky's and Papert's conclusions do not hold for multilayer perceptrons and other complex neural networks. The book gives background of modern neural network theory.

J. HOPFIELD, *Neural Networks and Physical Systems with Emergent Collective Computational Abilities*. This is a landmark paper (1982) in neural networks. It gives an algorithm for an asynchronous parallel processor, including associative memories from neurobiology (see chapter 4). This paper created interest in neural networks after the field lost its popularity in the 1960s. The reference is recommended for background because its neural network is a special instance of the modern theory developed in the text.

EXERCISES

1. Assume the minimum perceptible visual stimulus magnitude is 3×10^{-10} ergs. What is the approximate minimum number of photons the human eye can detect? Is the human brain a quantum measurement instrument?

2. Assuming the resolution at fovea with good contrast is about one minute of arc, how close is the human eye to the diffraction limit? Assuming diffraction limits optics, what is the approximate spacing of the photon detectors at fovea?

3. Assume the following:
- pulse frequency along axons = 100 Hz
- pulses needed to fire a neuron in each module = 2 to 5
- pulse propagation speed along axon = 100 m/s
- time to recognize an object = 0.5 s

Assuming at least one layer of neurons in each module, about how many modules in series are in human vision for initial recognition?

2

Neuron Physics and State Equations

This chapter presents the "standard model" for neurons. For the historian, the model's development is a rich story filled with false starts, theoretical preconceptions, and the interplay of personalities. The model's equations are the starting point to design systems and to understand human brain-mind functioning. This chapter summarizes the biological basis for the model in sufficient detail for understanding its derivation and—if needed—for refining it to depict the underlying biology more closely.

How sure are we that the standard model is reasonably correct? Will discoveries overthrow it and replace it with a significantly different model? Perhaps. In fact, section 2.4 discusses recent new research findings not yet part of the standard model.

If supplanted, however, the standard model will have played a valuable role because testing ideas and designing systems is respectable (though only in the last decade or so), especially since the national DARPA study [23] which surveyed the NN state of the art and identified applications.

Moreover, researchers commonly justify their programs with the standard model. Thus, the model gives a shared language allowing designers, researchers, and sponsors to appreciate and support each other. As seen in later chapters, the model also gives a powerful new tool to apply to real problems.

If researchers develop a better theory someday, it will probably be traced to results for improving the standard model.

2.1 NEURON STRUCTURE, PULSE GENERATION, AND PROPAGATION

The accepted human brain model is a system of 10^{10} to 10^{12} neurons of rather uniform material and structure. Studies show the neurons organized into about 200 modules with a few basic interneural kinds of signals. Groups of neurons with precise interconnections produce the systems and the functions of natural brain-minds. This section describes the traditional biochemical view of how a prototypical neuron functions in the central nervous system (CNS). It also introduces the basic language and gives a brief review of neurochemistry.

Summarizing [8,9,21,22,27,56], figure 2.1 shows a typical <u>neuron</u>. The neuron cell body, containing the nucleus and cytoplasm, is like other cells in basic structure and basic function. A neuron cell body differs from other cells because of the dendrites and axons.

<u>Dendrites</u> are branchlike protrusions from the neuron cell body. A typical cell has many. The receiving zones of impulses, called <u>synapses</u>, are on the cell body and dendrites. Some kinds of neuron have <u>spines</u> on the dendrites, thus creating more receiving sites.

An <u>axon</u>, the transmit channel of the impulses, is a long, fiberlike extension of the cell body. Each neuron has one axon, which branches or fans out to other neurons. The fan-out is typically 1:10,000 and more. The same signal, with varying time delays, propagates along each branch. Indeed, the large fan-out produces the brain's parallelism.

Each branch end has a synapse. A typical synapse is a bulblike structure at the end of an axon branch. The synapses are on the cell body, dendrites, and spines, shown in figure 2.2. There may be 10^4 to 10^5 synapses on a neuron.

Between the synapse and the target neuron is a narrow gap, typically 20 nanometers wide. Special molecules called <u>neurotransmitters</u> cross the synaptic gap to receptor sites on the target neuron. The flow of neurotransmitter molecules is the transmission of signals between synapse and neuron.

The signals from a neuron are inhibitory or excitatory, not both. Excitatory signals tend to fire the target neuron; inhibitory signals tend to prevent firing. A neuron fires, that is, sends a signal along its axon, depending on the time-integrated effect of all signals crossing its synaptic gaps.

Moreover, each neuron sends only one kind of signal. That is, a neuron cannot be excitatory to some target neurons and inhibitory to others. (Recent studies show that some neurons in the retina may be excitatory and inhibitory, but they are the only known exceptions [69].)

An electrochemical mechanism produces and propagates signals along the axon. At equilibrium (no signaling) the interior of the neuron and its axon is negative relative to the exterior because the interior has an excess of negative ions, while the exterior has an excess of positive ions. The negative ions are Cl^-, PhO^-, and carbon–oxygen acids. The positive ions are Na^+, K^+, Ca^+, and Mg^+.

A biological ion pump, powered by mitochondria, causes the ion concentrations in and around the neuron. <u>Mitochondria</u> are structures in the neuron using and transferring the energy produced by burning fuel (sugar) and molecular oxygen. In a sense, mitochondria are microscopic energy sources.

The excess of positive and negative charges generates an electric field across the neuron surface, shown in figure 2.3. The plasma membrane of the neuron holds the charges

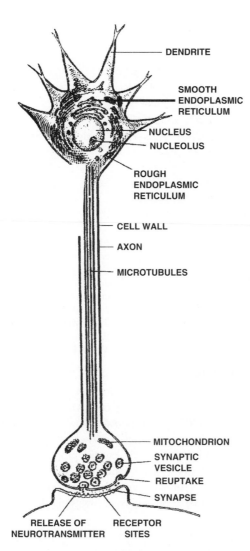

Figure 2.1 Structure of a typical mammalian neuron. A neuron functions metabolically like other cells. It has a single long axon from the cell body to the synapses. Dendrites are outgrowths of the cell body and form synapses with other neurons. (Figure 2.2 shows more detail.) The synaptic terminal stores neurotransmitters in vesicles. Microtubules provide structural rigidity and transport material along the axon. (From Bloom, et al. *Brain, Mind and Behavior*. Reprinted by permission of W. H. Freeman and Co., 1985.)

apart. The membrane is selective to diffusion of particular molecules, and its diffusion selectivity varies with time and length along the axon. Indeed, varying the membrane diffusivity produces and propagates signal pulses along the axon and across the synaptic gaps.

The axon signal pulses, also called action potentials, are described electrically by current-voltage characteristics, shown in figure 2.4. Injecting a current pulse into the axon causes the potential across the membrane to vary. Chemical signals at excitatory synapses inject current into the axon. As described next, the current pulses stimulate an excitatory neuron to fire.

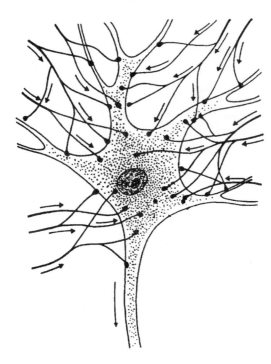

Figure 2.2   A neuron may be
connected with others by tens of
thousands of synaptic contacts on its
dendrites and cell body. The synaptic
contacts are small compared with the
cell body. (From The Diagram Group.
The Brain—A User's Manual.
Reprinted by permission of Diagram
Visual Information Limited, 1987.)

The equilibrium potential of the axon is about -70 mV. When injected with an inhibitory (hyperpolarization) signal pulse, the response is a RC-type, that is exponential, followed by relaxation to equilibrium. When injected with a small excitatory pulse (depolarization), the response is also a RC-type response followed by relaxation.

When the injection current causes the voltage to exceed threshold (typically -40 mV), the potential rapidly continues to rise. Thus, the current produces a single pulse with a peak-to-peak amplitude of about 120 mV and a duration of 1 ms.

A pulse, caused by injected current, propagates without weakening along all branches of the axon. A complex, not fully understood sequence involving the ions maintains the pulse shape and strength.

A brief description of the production and propagation of a pulse by a step-by-step electrochemical process follows, and is also shown in figure 2.5.

1. Chemical signals at excitatory synapses inject current in the axon.
2. Rising positive charges in the cell trigger Na^+ gates along the membrane to open (threshold about -40 mV).
3. An influx of Na^+ causes the interior to go positive ($+60$ mV). The influx is caused by the electrical potential and the concentration gradients.
4. The positive interior causes adjacent Na^+ gates to open so that an impulse propagates down the axon. The propagating speed is 0.5 m/s to 120 m/s depending on the axon diameter. (For example, during each pulse in a 1-μm diameter squid axon, about 3 picomoles of Na per cm^2 enter the axon.)

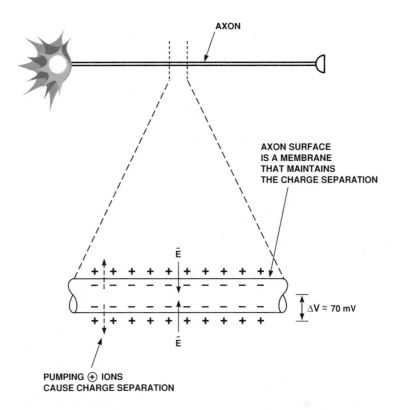

Figure 2.3   The movement of electrically charged ions across the neuron's cell wall membrane produces the pulses along an axon. At equilibrium a neuron has a net negative charge inside and a net positive charge outside caused by the pumping of sodium and potassium ions (sodium outward, potassium inward). The charges produce an inward-directed electrical field and a voltage potential of about -60 to -75 mV.

5. The Na^+ gates close by the outflow of K^+ from the interior.

6. Na collects in the interior from each pulse while the exterior loses K. The recovery to equilibrium is by a Na-K exchange process.

The Na-K exchange, or pump, is driven by the hydrolysis of adenosine triphosphate (ATP). ATP is widely used in nature to furnish energy for chemical reactions. ATP spontaneously goes to adenosine diphosphate (ADP) and inorganic phosphate (P_i) by hydrolysis with the release of 30 kJ/mol. That is

$$ATP \rightarrow ADP + P_i \text{ (release 30 kJ/mol)}.$$

This energy can be used to drive a biochemical reaction that might not normally proceed. For example, consider the reaction $X \rightarrow Y$ for which 20 kJ/mol must be supplied under standard conditions. If the conversion of X to Y is coupled to ATP hydrolysis, the combined reaction would be

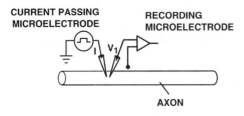

CURRENT PASSING
MICROELECTRODE

RECORDING
MICROELECTRODE

V_1

AXON

CURRENT PULSES THROUGH ELECTRODE I

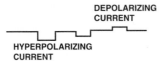

DEPOLARIZING
CURRENT

HYPERPOLARIZING
CURRENT

RECORDING FROM MICROELECTRODE V_1

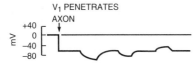

V_1 PENETRATES
AXON

+40
0
−40
−80

mV

TWO DEPOLARIZING CURRENT PULSES
THROUGH ELECTRODE I

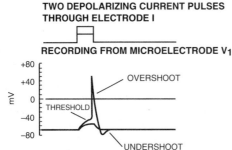

RECORDING FROM MICROELECTRODE V_1

+80
+40
0
−40
−80

mV

OVERSHOOT

THRESHOLD

UNDERSHOOT

Figure 2.4   Axon current-voltage characteristics. Injecting a negative current pulse (hyperpolarization) into an axon at equilibrium causes a RC-type of response. Injecting a small positive current pulse (depolarization) also causes a RC-kind of response. Injecting a depolarizing current so that the voltage exceeds a threshold causes a pulse with an amplitude of about 120 mV and a duration of about 1 ms. (From Kuffler, et al. *From Neuron to Brain*. Adapted by permission of Sinauer Associates, Inc., 1984).

$$ATP + X \rightarrow ADP + P_i + Y \text{ (release 10 kJ/mol)}.$$

Under standard conditions the reaction proceeds spontaneously.

Many versions of the Na-K pump are energetically plausible, and it remains to be determined which version occurs in living cells.

Summarizing [28], a proposed model for the Na-K pump is the following sequence.

1. Exterior reactions:

$$K^+ + \text{protein} \rightarrow \text{protein}-K^+$$

The protein$-K^+$ diffuses to the interior by a concentration gradient.

2. Interior reactions:

$$ATP + \text{protein}-K^+ + Na^+ \rightarrow ADP + K^+ + \text{phosphoprotein}-Na^+$$

The phosphoprotein$-Na^+$ complex diffuses to the exterior by a concentration gradient.

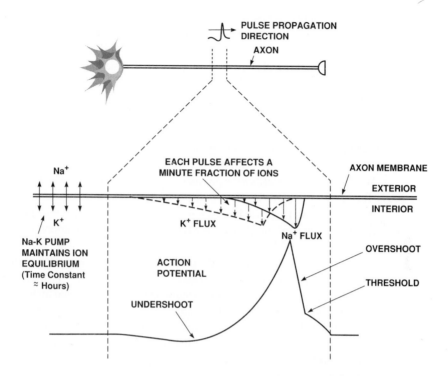

Figure 2.5   Process for generating a pulse in an axon. Sodium and potassium channels cover the axon membrane. At equilibrium the channels are closed. When a depolarization voltage exceeds threshold the channels open for about 1 ms during which time about 6000 sodium ions pass. The flow of ions causes a pulse, and the axon voltage goes from about −70 mV to +50 mV. The channels then close spontaneously and recovery to equilibrium occurs by an energy-driven ion pump, which is also part of the membrane.

3. Exterior reactions:

$$\text{phosphoprotein}-\text{Na}^+ \rightarrow \text{Na}^+ + \text{protein}$$

This last reaction takes place because of an enzyme.

The pump model assumes a carrier protein molecule shuttling back and forth across the membrane, transporting K^+ on the inward trip and Na^+ on the outward trip. Movement of the carrier-passenger complex is driven by a concentration gradient, this gradient being determined by the state of the phosphorylation of the carrier.

In comparison, [22] describes another pump model. In this model, a large protein molecule (mol. wt. = 120,000), called Na^+K^+-ATPase, is oriented in the membrane with part of the protein exposed at other faces. The protein neither rotates nor shuttles back and forth. Three Na^+ ions bind to sites on the inner surface, and two K^+ ions bind to sites on the outer surface. The protein then undergoes a conformational change and the three Na^+

ions are pumped outward, possibly by the creation of a channel. The two K^+ ions are then moved inward, by another conformational change, back to the original shape.

The Na-K pump has been studied in detail because of its importance. The mechanism, however, for transporting Na^+ out of and K^+ into the membrane is not known in detail, although most researchers now believe that conformational changes in the Na-K-ATPase enable the ion movements.

The above description of a propagating axon pulse assumes a smooth, uniform axon surface. In fact a sheath of myelin with gaps along its length frequently encloses many axons. The basic mechanism, however, still holds. With myelin sheaths, the pulse propagates by jumping from gap to gap along the axon, resulting in higher propagation speeds.

While the model describes the production and propagation of a single pulse, one pulse does not carry information. In fact, many processes produce pulses randomly.

Research shows that encoding of information is by the frequency of the pulse train, a process called frequency shift keying (FSK) in digital communications. The frequency is in the range of 10 to 100 Hz.

An example of neural FSK is in the measurement of muscle motion. Muscle spindles, a kind of sensor, measure the rate and extent of muscle stretch. As shown in figure 2.6, mechanical motion leads to local depolarization in the nerve terminal by locally decreasing the electrical field. The depolarization, equivalent to a current injection, causes a train of impulses along the axon when currents exceed the threshold. The frequency of the impulses is proportional to the depolarization. In turn, depolarization is proportional to the mechanical movement. Thus, the pulse train frequency encodes the signal that measures the muscle motion.

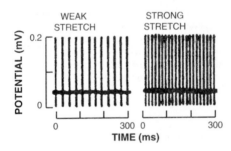

Figure 2.6   Pulse trains produced by stretching muscles. A sensory nerve responds to the stretching of a muscle by firing at a rate proportional to the stretch. (From Kuffler, et al. *From Neuron to Brain*. Reprinted by permission of Sinauer Associates, Inc., 1984.)

When a pulse train signal reaches a synapse, synaptic transmission transfers the signal to the target neuron. Synaptic transmission is the chemical transfer of signals from one neuron to another across the synaptic gap. The signaling is an extension of nerve impulse transmission and membrane potential characteristics. While direct electrical interactions among neighboring neurons is possible, chemical transmission is the dominant mechanism of signaling among neurons.

Synaptic transmission raises two main questions: How do neurotransmitters act on the postsynaptic neuron to produce excitation and inhibition? How does the presynaptic terminal release the neurotransmitters?

Figure 2.7 shows the prototypical model of a synapse.

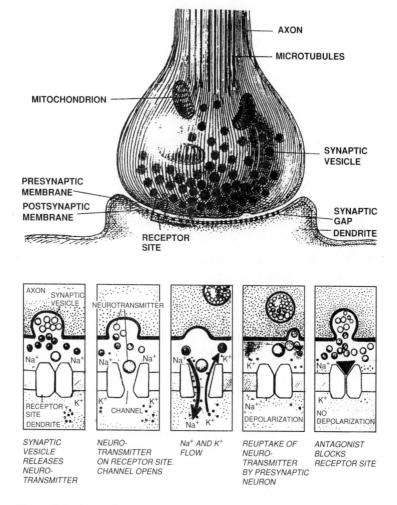

Figure 2.7   A step-by-step sequence of neurotransmitter release and recovery (reuptake) at a hypothetical synapse. (From Bloom, et al. *Brain, Mind and Behavior*. Reprinted by permission of W. H. Freeman and Co., 1985.)

Starting with the first question, increasing the permeability to Na^+ and K^+ of the post-junctional membrane produces synaptic excitation, leading to a depolarizing synaptic potential. Excitation results from driving the membrane potential over threshold. A common excitatory neurotransmitter is acetylcholine (ACh).

Summarizing [56], the sequence for synaptic excitation by ACh is as follows.

1. Presynapse sites release ACh^+ (see below).
2. ACh^+ diffuses across the synaptic gap to the postsynaptic membrane.
3. The postsynaptic membrane permeability to Na^+ and K^+ greatly increases.

4. Na$^+$ and K$^+$ ion currents across the membrane drive the potential in the target neuron to the -20 mV-to-0 mV range. A large amplifying mechanism takes place because one ACh$^+$ ion causes about 1000 Na$^+$/K$^+$ ions to cross the membrane.

Increasing the permeability to Cl$^-$ and K$^+$ of the post-junctional membrane produces synaptic inhibition, leading to a hyperpolarizing synaptic potential. Driving the membrane potential away from threshold gives inhibition. Inhibitory neurotransmitters are mainly unknown; however, one identified inhibitory neurotransmitter is γ-aminobutyric acid (GABA).

The sequence for synaptic inhibition is as follows.

1. Presynapse sites release an inhibitory neurotransmitter (see below).
2. The neurotransmitter diffuses across the synaptic gap to the postsynaptic membrane.
3. The postsynaptic membrane permeability to Cl$^-$ and K$^+$ greatly increases.
4. Cl$^-$ and K$^+$ ion currents across the membrane drive the potential of the target neuron below -70 mV.

The differences in excitation and inhibition are primarily membrane permeability differences. Inhibition, however, is difficult to account for by changes only in postsynaptic permeability.

Figure 2.8 shows an axoaxonic synapse where an inhibitory synapse goes to the presynaptic junction of an excitatory synapse. Researchers have found, by electron microscopy, axoaxonic synapses at many locations in the mammalian CNS. (NN modeling rarely assumes axoaxonic mechanisms.)

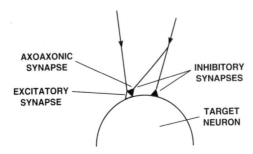

Figure 2.8 Presynaptic inhibition. An excitatory synapse is affected by an inhibitory axoaxonic synapse. The effect is to reduce the neurotransmitter quanta released from the excitatory terminal.

Presynaptic inhibition is helpful when many pathways converge because the system can selectively suppress inputs. The selection cannot be done by postsynaptic conductance, which changes the whole target cell. Researchers do not know the relative importance of presynaptic and postsynaptic inhibition in the CNS.

Considering the second question of presynaptic release, the release of neurotransmitters in the synaptic gap is a complex process. Observations show that an action potential pulse in the presynaptic fiber normally gives rise, after a delay, to a large depolarizing potential in the postsynaptic membrane. The depolarizing potential usually reaches threshold and produces an action potential.

Figure 2.9 shows the presynaptic and postsynaptic potentials. The maximum excitatory postsynaptic potential (epsp) is related to the maximum presynaptic potential. The delay time is sensitive to temperature. For example, squid neuron results show delay times varying from 0.5 ms at 20° C to 7 ms at 2° C.

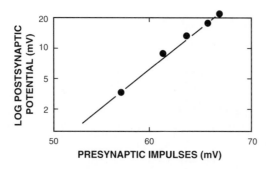

Figure 2.9 The relation between excitatory presynaptic and excitatory postsynaptic potential (epsp). (From Kuffler, et al. *From Neuron to Brain.* Adapted by permission of Sinauer Associates, Inc., 1984.)

Another finding is that removing calcium or adding magnesium to the presynaptic junction reduces the neurotransmitter ACh release. Research shows that the release of neurotransmitter ACh^+ is in quanta having about 1000 molecules of ACh^+. Although the quanta may vary, research shows fixed molecules per quanta. (For example, neuromuscular synapses have about 200 quanta per release.) In general, the quanta per release depends on the neuron and varies widely. Finally, at low Ca concentration, releases have only a few quanta.

The origin and targets of nerve fibers establish information and meaning because signals are similar in all nerve cells. That is, meaning has to do with the particular neural group, while frequency coding conveys information about the stimulus intensity. Thus, precise connections among selected neurons produce the wealth of information reaching us in the visual and other sensory systems.

Learning is connected to synaptic processes. Learning correlates to and is affected by synaptic efficacy, which has to do with neurotransmitter release. The efficacy is caused by changes in the quanta per release, not the molecules per quanta. Trains of impulses can lead to a continuing rise in the response. The rise, called <u>facilitation</u>, is caused by increases in the quanta released by the presynaptic terminal. Figure 2.10 shows facilitation graphically. Presynaptic inhibition, on the other hand, reduces the quanta released from the affected terminal.

Learning also affects the shape of the synapses. The presynaptic cavities change from a triangular cross section to a rounded cross section. Research shows that the cross-section change is permanent.

Moreover, learning affects the number of synapses on the neurons, especially during the early years of life. In the developing brain, the synapses to each neuron grow to a maximum at about age two in human beings. Between ages two and seven the number of synapses reduces about one-half. The drop is during the intense learning of basic skills. After age seven, the neuron population remains nearly constant until shortly before death.

Many studies show relationships between talent and neuron structure. In general, research shows more dendrites associated with talent. For example, an expert pianist has a more complex dendritic structure in the motor system than the average person.

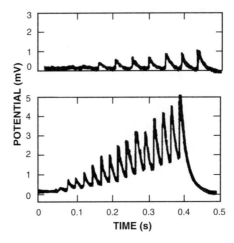

Figure 2.10 Facilitation caused by increased quanta release. Changes in synaptic efficacy are usually caused by changes in quanta content of neurotransmitters. The progressive increase in transmitter release is believed related to increases in calcium in the presynaptic terminal. (From Kuffler, et al. *From Neuron to Brain*. Reprinted by permission of Sinauer Associates, Inc., 1984.)

Other nonneural structures also play a part in overall functioning. For example, measurements show that samples of the frontal lobe of Einstein's brain had more glial cells per neuron than average. (The glial cells are support cells of the brain and greatly outnumber neurons.)

In summary, the traditional view of neural functioning provides a basis for the standard NN model, presented next. The standard model gives powerful insights into human brain-mind thought processes, shown in later chapters. Section 2.4 summarizes recent findings not yet in the standard model.

2.2 NEURON STATE EQUATIONS

Early NN researchers formulated equations describing biological nervous systems primarily from the emergent behavior of interconnected elementary units (neurons) rather than from detailed modeling of neural mechanisms, such as the Hodgkin–Huxley system [47]. Although it is well known that a neuron transmits voltage spikes along its axon, many studies show that the effects on the receiving neurons can be usefully summarized by voltage potentials in the neuron interior that vary slowly and continuously during the time scale of a single spike. That is, the time scale of the interior neuron potential is long compared to the spike duration. The standard NN equations reflect this viewpoint.

Assume a neuron interacting with other neurons and outside stimuli, shown in figure 2.11. Denoting the ith neuron by ν_i, the model starts by defining two variables, x_i and Z_{ij}, which describe the neuron's state.

One state variable of ν_i is x_i, where

$$x_i(t) = \text{activation level of the ith neuron.}$$

Or (physiological view),

$$x_i(t) = \text{deviation of neuron potential from equilibrium [volts].}$$

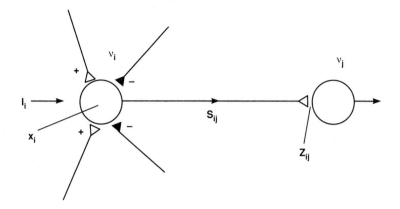

Figure 2.11   Schematic diagram of a neuron and a neural network. (a) Neuron, v_i, with potential, x_i relative to equilibrium, sends a signal, S_{ij}, along the axon to a target neuron, v_j. The signal affects the target neuron with a coupling strength, Z_{ij}. The signal may be excitatory ($Z_{ij} > 0$) or inhibitory ($Z_{ij} < 0$). Other inputs, I_i, to the neuron model external stimuli. (b) Interconnections of many neurons form a neural network, which approximates the signal processing of biological nervous systems.

Or (psychological view),

$$x_i(t) = \underline{\text{short-term memory}} \text{ (STM) trace.}$$

The second state variable, Z_{ij}, is associated with v_i's interaction with v_j (another neuron), where

$$Z_{ij}(t) = \text{synaptic coupling coefficient.}$$

Or (physiological view),

$$Z_{ij}(t) = \text{neurotransmitter average release rate per unit axon signal}$$
$$\text{frequency [volts/sec/Hz} = \text{volts].}$$

Or (psychological view),

$$Z_{ij}(t) = \underline{\text{long-term memory}} \text{ (LTM) trace.}$$

Four models for the STM and LTM traces are

1. Additive STM equation

2. Passive decay LTM equation

3. Shunting STM equation

4. Extended LTM equation

In practice, the model selected depends on the application.

1. Additive STM equation. To formulate a set of ordinary differential equations for $x_i(t)$ and $\overline{Z_{ij}(t)}$, assume a change in neuron potential from equilibrium ($-70\,\text{mV}$). In general the change is caused by internal and external processes.

$$\frac{dx_i}{dt} = \left(\frac{dx_i}{dt}\right)_{internal} + \left(\frac{dx_i}{dt}\right)_{external} , \quad \forall i. \tag{2.1}$$

Assume inputs from other neurons and stimuli are additive (agrees with many experiments).

$$\frac{dx_i}{dt} = \left(\frac{dx_i}{dt}\right)_{internal} + \left(\frac{dx_i}{dt}\right)_{excitatory} - \left(\frac{dx_i}{dt}\right)_{inhibitory} + \left(\frac{dx_i}{dt}\right)_{stimuli} , \quad \forall i. \tag{2.2}$$

Assume the internal neuron processes are stable.

$$\left(\frac{dx_i}{dt}\right)_{internal} = -A_i(x_i)x_i, \quad A_i(x_i) > 0, \; \forall i. \tag{2.3}$$

Assume additive synaptic excitation proportional to the pulse train frequency.

$$\left(\frac{dx_i}{dt}\right)_{excitatory} \propto \sum_{\substack{other \\ neurons}} (\text{average axon frequency}) (\text{synaptic coupling coefficient}). \tag{2.4}$$

Or,

$$\left(\frac{dx_i}{dt}\right)_{excitatory} = \sum_{\substack{k=1 \\ k\neq i}}^{n} S_{ki} Z_{ki}, \; \forall i. \tag{2.5}$$

The phrase "Z_{ki} gates S_{ki}" describes the term $S_{ki} Z_{ki}$, where S_{ki} = frequency of signal in the $v_k \to v_i$ axon evaluated at v_i.

In general, S_{ki}, called the signal function, depends on the propagation time delay from v_k to v_i (τ_{ki}) and the threshold for firing of v_k (Γ_k). Formally,

$$S_{ki}(t) = S_{ki}[x_k(t - \tau_{ki}) - \Gamma_k] \geq 0. \tag{2.6}$$

S_{ki} is referred to in two ways depending on the situation:

$$S_{ki} = \begin{cases} \text{Sampling signal when considered input, or} \\ \text{Performance signal when considered output.} \end{cases}$$

Figure 2.12 shows the following three common signal functions:
Piecewise linear signal function,

$$S_{ki}(t) = b_{ki} f[x_k(t - \tau_{ki}) - \Gamma_{ki}]^+, \tag{2.7}$$

where

$$[x_i]^+ = \max\{0, x_i\}. \tag{2.8}$$

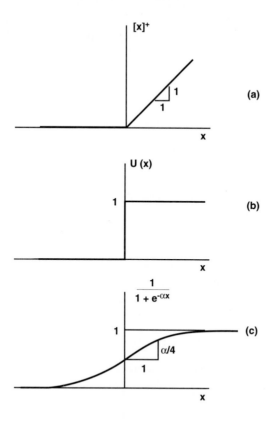

Figure 2.12   Common neural network signal functions. (a) A piecewise linear function models the nonlinear off-on characteristic of neurons. (b) A step function gives the abrupt off-on characteristic and a maximum output. (c) A sigmoid function models the off-on, nonlinear, smooth, and bounded characteristics. The abruptness is set by the slope near zero. Other signal functions are possible.

Step function signal function,

$$S_{ki}(t) = U[x_i] = \begin{cases} 0 & \text{if } x_i < 0 \\ 1 & \text{otherwise.} \end{cases} \tag{2.9}$$

Sigmoid function signal function,

$$S_{ki}(t) = b_{ki}\, f[x_k(t - \tau_{ki}) - \Gamma_{ki}],\ b_{ki} \geq 0, \tag{2.10}$$

where, for example,

$$f(x) = \frac{1}{1 + e^{-\alpha x}}. \tag{2.11}$$

Other signal functions are also possible. Moreover, many global NN properties are only weakly dependent on the particular signal function. Some NN properties, however, are dependent on the signal function (see section 4.1).

Assume hardwiring of the inhibitory inputs from other neurons, that is, their coupling strength, or effectiveness, is constant. Then,

$$\left(\frac{dx_i}{dt}\right)_{inhibitory} = \sum_{\substack{k=1 \\ k\neq i}}^{n} C_{ki},\ C_{ki} \geq 0,\ \forall i, \tag{2.12}$$

where

$$C_{ki}(t) = c_{ki} g[x_k(t - \tau_{ki}) - \Gamma_k], \; c_{ki} \geq 0 \tag{2.13}$$

and $g[\;]$ is a sigmoid or a piecewise linear function.

2. Passive decay LTM equation. Assume the excitatory coupling strength varies with time. A common model is

$$\frac{dZ_{ij}}{dt} = -B_{ij}(Z_{ij})Z_{ij} + S'_{ij}[x_j]^+, \; \forall i, j. \tag{2.14}$$

S'_{ij} is like S_{ij}, but it may differ in presynaptic dependency on x_i. Assume

$$S'_{ki}(t) = b'_{ki} f[x_k(t - \tau_{ki}) - \Gamma_{ki}]^+, \; \forall k, i. \tag{2.15}$$

The term $S'_{ij}[x_j]^+$ in (2.14) shows that to increase Z_{ij}, v_i must send a signal S'_{ij} to v_j and at the same time v_j be activated ($x_j > 0$).

Note that the STM and LTM equations are not solvable until specifying a set of coefficients, A_i, S_{ki}, C_{ki}, B_{ij}, S'_{ij}, and until giving the external stimuli $I_i(t)$.

3. Shunting STM equation. The shunting STM equation is a better model of the neuron physics than the additive STM equation; however, it is more complex. Consider an equivalent electrical circuit for the membrane, shown in figure 2.13. The equation for this circuit is

$$C\frac{\partial V}{\partial t} = (V^+ - V)g^+ + (V^- - V)g^- + (V^P - V)g^P, \tag{2.16}$$

where figure 2.13 defines $V(t)$, V^+, V^-, and V^P. Assume

$$\left. \begin{array}{ll} V^- \leq V(t) & \leq V^+ \\ V^- \leq V^P & < V^+ \\ V^- - V^P & << V^+ - V^P \end{array} \right\} \tag{2.17}$$

The circuit relaxes from an initial value to a final value depending on the three right-hand terms in (2.16).

For example, first assume $V(0) = V^P$. Then, for g^+, $g^P = 0$, the system goes from V^P to V^+. Second, for g^+, $g^P = 0$, it then relaxes from V^+ to V^-. Third, for g^+, $g^- = 0$, it relaxes from V^- to V^P (equilibrium).

The membrane equation approximates the action potential in an axon, shown in figure 2.14.

The shunting STM equation starts by defining the following variables. Let

$$\left. \begin{array}{l} V(t) = x_i \\ V^+ = B_i \\ V^- = -D_i \\ V^P = 0 \\ g^+ = I_i + \sum_{k \neq i} S_{ki} Z_{ki}^{(+)} \\ g^- = J_i + \sum_{l \neq i} S_{li} Z_{li}^{(-)} \\ g^P = A \\ C = 1 \end{array} \right\} \tag{2.18}$$

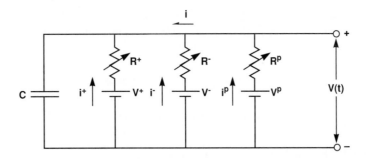

Figure 2.13   Circuit analogy for a neuron membrane. V^+, V^-, V^p are the maximum, minimum, and equilibrium voltages, respectively, inside a neuron. The voltages act like batteries in an electrical circuit. They produce a fluctuating output voltage, $V(t)$, representing the action potential inside the neuron. The membrane model leads to the shunting STM equation.

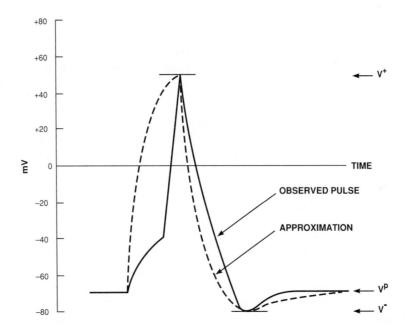

Figure 2.14   Action potential and its approximation. Proper selection of the circuit parameters (see figure 2.13), C, R^+, R^-, R^p, gives a pulse shape that approximates a biological neuron pulse.

Substituting (2.18) in (2.16) gives the shunting STM equation,

$$\dot{x}_i = -A_i x_i + (B_i - x_i)[\sum_{k \neq i} S_{ki} Z_{ki}^{(+)} + I_i]$$

$$-(x_i + D_i)[\sum_{l \neq i} S_{li} Z_{li}^{(-)} + J_i], \ \forall i. \qquad (2.19)$$

4. Extended LTM equation. The passive decay LTM equation does not explicitly model the neurotransmitter level needed for some applications. For these applications, redefine some of the variables as follows.

Let

$$Z_{ki} = \text{usable excitatory neurotransmitter level [moles]},$$

and

$$M_{ki} = \text{maximum excitatory neurotransmitter level [moles]},$$
$$\text{(the LTM trace in this case)}.$$

Model the usable neurotransmitter level by

$$\dot{Z}_{ki} = K(M_{ki} - Z_{ki}) - C S'_{ki} Z_{ki}, \ K > C, \ \forall i, k. \tag{2.20}$$

Model the LTM trace by

$$\dot{M}_{ki} = -\beta M_{ki} + S''_{ki}[x_i]^+, \ \forall i, k. \tag{2.21}$$

Examination of (2.20) and (2.21) gives the following characteristics. Without signals on an axon, the neurotransmitter level, Z_{ki}, rises at rate K to a maximum level, M_{ki}, (modeling reuptake of the neurotransmitters). The second right-hand term in (2.20) shows that axon signals deplete the neurotransmitter at rate C. Experimentally K is somewhat larger than C.

Note that for long time intervals, x_i is proportional to Z_{ki}, by the STM equation. By the LTM equation, x_i is also proportional to M_{ki}. Or, M_{ki} is proportional to Z_{ki}.

Thus, the simple passive decay LTM equation corresponds to long times. To study short-term effects, however, requires using the more realistic extended three-variable LTM model.

2.3 NETWORK EQUATIONS

Interactions among neurons are generally nonlinear, chiefly because of the signal function. In principle, the nonlinear differential equations that describe the STM trace and LTM trace of a group of neurons can be solved. In practice, except for the simplest cases, the equations are intractable, and researchers must apply other approaches.

Using a single node to represent a pool of interacting neurons is often convenient. Figure 2.15 shows a typical situation consisting of a group of neurons and one output node. In the group,

$$\dot{x}_i = -A_i x_i + \sum_{k \neq i}^{N} S_{ki} Z_{ki} - \sum_{l \neq i,k}^{N} C_{li} + I_i, \ \forall i, \tag{2.22}$$

and

$$\dot{Z}_{ij} = -B_{ij} Z_{ij} + S'_{ij}[x_j]^+, \ \forall i, j, \tag{2.23}$$

where the summation indices reflect the interconnections.

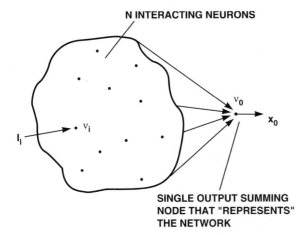

N INTERACTING NEURONS

ν_0

x_0

ν_i

I_i

SINGLE OUTPUT SUMMING
NODE THAT "REPRESENTS"
THE NETWORK

Figure 2.15   If the time scales of the input and neuron dynamics are properly chosen, a single neuron, ν_0, may represent a group of neurons. In this interpretation, the activation level of ν_0 is proportional to the fraction of excited neurons in the group.

At the output node,

$$\dot{x}_0 = -A_0 x_0 + \sum_{i=1}^{N} S_{i0} Z_{i0} + I_0 \tag{2.24}$$

and

$$\dot{Z}_{i0} = -B_{i0} Z_{i0} + S'_{i0}[x_0]^+, \ \forall i. \tag{2.25}$$

With assumptions, x_0 is proportional to the number of excited neurons in the pool. For example, let

$$\left. \begin{array}{l} Z_{i0} \approx \text{constant (slowly varying)}, \ \forall i, \\[1ex] S_{i0} \approx s_{i0}[x_i]^+ \ (\text{short delays, low thresholds}, \ \forall i). \end{array} \right\} \tag{2.26}$$

Then (2.24) becomes

$$\dot{x}_0 = -A_0 x_o + \sum_{i=1}^{N} s_{i0}[x_i]^+ Z_{i0} + I_0. \tag{2.27}$$

If A_0 is large and the time scales for integrating inputs in (2.24) are short, x_0 is proportional to the number of excited nodes in the pool as $t \to \infty$.

The preceding example leads to a formulation for groups of neurons.

Consider groups of interacting neurons $\{\nu_1, \nu_2,...\}$. Let x_i be redefined to be

$$x_i = \text{ potentials of cell populations in group } \nu_i.$$

Assume ν_i has B excitable sites, with x_i sites excited and B-x_i sites unexcited. This is a binary model, that is, the neurons are on or off.

The shunting STM equation then gives

$$\dot{x}_i = -A_i x_i + (B_i - x_i)[\sum_{k \neq i} S_{ki} Z_{ki}^{(+)} + I_i]$$
$$- (x_i + D_i)[\sum_{l \neq i} S_{li} Z_{li}^{(-)} + J_i], \forall i. \tag{2.28}$$

Assuming certain terms negligible gives

$$\dot{x}_i = -A_i x_i + (B_i - x_i) I_i - x_i \sum_{k \neq i} I_k, \forall i. \tag{2.29}$$

Thus, the state equations for a single neuron have the same form as that for a group of interacting neurons. With this interpretation, x_i is the excited state in a group. For a group, however, $A_i = A_i(x_i)$ and thus is not constant.

The two interpretations of x_i —excitation of a neuron or excited neurons in a group— may cause confusion. The application must carefully state the interpretation. The following chapters apply both interpretations.

2.4 RECENT NEURAL-BIOLOGY FINDINGS

Section 2.1 describes the traditional biochemical view of a prototypical neuron in the CNS. The NN models, derived in sections 2.2 and 2.3, reflect this view. Recent findings in the brain sciences, however, have altered the traditional view. Most of this new information, outlined below, remains to be incorporated into NN models. Undoubtedly, future NN models will contain some of the new findings.

To summarize for perspective, in the traditional view of a CNS neuron, particular molecules function as neurotransmitters and charge-carriers in membrane ion channels. The movement of these molecules is the mechanism for the millisecond-to-millisecond communication in the brain-mind.

The prototypical neurotransmitters are the catecholamines (CA), studied since 1905. These are 3,4 dihydroxy derivatives of phenylephyamine, occurring in the brainstem nuclei and elsewhere, which enable mental functioning. Section 2.1 describes the synthesis, storage, release, receptor interaction, and action termination of neurotransmitters.

In the traditional view, starting with the pioneering work of Hebb (1949), a biology theory relates synaptic function to learning and memory. In this theory, a neuron is not a simple digital switch as envisioned by McCulloch and Pitts [66]. That is, the internal cellular environment, the local external cellular environment, and distance regulation by hormones affect synaptic functioning.

Moreover, in the traditional model, presynaptic activity causes postsynaptic receptor activity and ion fluxes, resulting in permanent changes of the synaptic structure, which in turn alter function. The structural changes are changes of the postsynaptic density (PSD), a protein layer in the synaptic gap that anchors the receptors. Changes in the PSD shape expose formerly hidden receptors and alter the electrical properties of the synapse. An example is the NMDA receptors of the neurotransmitter glutamate in synaptic spines of hippocampal neurons [62].

This is the traditional biochemical view of neural functioning. It gives the most useful model for molecular-physiologic-behavior interactions (see chapter 8). Nevertheless, new findings, especially in the last five years, are rapidly altering this view in significant ways.

Recent research [8] strongly suggests that the human brain-mind has a control hierarchy of modules among many levels of organization. The hierarchy is the whole brain, neural groups, neurons, synapses, molecules, and genes. A basic finding is that the CNS reacts to external stimuli at all levels of organization down to the genome in a well-defined cascade of biochemical processes.

Moreover, a stimulus alters functioning throughout this hierarchy on a millisecond time scale. That is, stimuli—such as stress—affect the rate of gene readout in brain cells on a millisecond time scale!

Another finding is that neurons commonly use more than one kind of neurotransmitter and that the kind of neurotransmitter may change over time, giving another mechanism for memory and learning. The traditional view of synapses with a single kind of neurotransmitter is being refined and extended to the view of multiple transmitters at each synapse.

Another finding is that receptors also occur on the presynaptic junction. The presynaptic receptors give a negative feedback mechanism.

The implications of these findings, for which a detailed description is beyond the scope of the text, are enormous and profound.

For example, the connectionist view that knowledge lies in the synapses is too restrictive and ignores molecular and genome processes. The functionalism view that mental activity is, in principle, possible in many media is not supported by the physical evidence. The brain-mind has no hardware-software partitioning, and basic biochemical processes intimately root cognition to the genome level. On the other hand, the extreme reductionist view that complete knowledge of the genome and the molecular physics is sufficient, ignores the cases of, say, genetically identical aquatic fleas with different nervous systems.

Thus, both genetic and molecular knowledge is necessary to understand mechanisms; by themselves they are insufficient.

Indeed, an emerging view of brain-mind functioning is that of neural dynamics across many levels of organization on a millisecond time scale, and that learning is caused by altered synaptic structures <u>and</u> by altered DNA readout. Current research in the life sciences is becoming focused on defining the control levels and delineating the rules of interaction among the levels.

Chapters 8 and 9 return to NN models of complex and higher cognitive processes.

SUGGESTED REFERENCES

R. KEYNES, *Ion Channels in the Nerve-Cell Membrane*. This short article describes the generation of nerve impulses by the flow of sodium and potassium ions across the nerve membrane. The article is a good overview reference before reading Kuffler.

S. KUFFLER, J. NICHOLLS, AND R. MARTIN, *From Neuron to Brain*. The book describes the chemistry of neuron signal production and transmission. It gives information on the action potentials, ion concentrations, and experimental techniques. Portions of chapters 4 through 12 are the closest to the text. The writing is from an experimental biology point of view.

E. KANDEL AND J. SCHWARTZ, *Principles of Neural Science*. This book is an introductory text for students of biology, behavior, and medicine. It treats neuroanatomy extensively. The book is the most complete reference widely available and is simpler than Kuffler. The book is not mathematical.

A. REES AND M. STERNBERG, *From Cells to Atoms*. This book is an introduction to molecular biology. The illustrated format makes the book a worthwhile introduction to molecular biology for the beginner. It is also a summary for the mature student.

E. DUPRAW, *Cell and Molecular Biology*. The literature of molecular biology is extensive. This book is a textbook for senior undergraduates and graduate students. Chapter 3 discusses the biochemistry of energy transfer. The text material on ATP hydrolysis is from this chapter.

J. DARNELL, H. LODISH, AND D. BALTIMORE, *Molecular Biology*. This is a formiable textbook on molecular biology at the intermediate level that can be read for background for the kind of graduate course for which the present text is designed. Chapter 15 describes the Na-K pump.

I. BLACK, *Information in the Brain*. This little book gives a remarkably complete synthesis of neuro-science from a molecular prespective. Chapter 2 summarizes the traditional biochemical view of the synapse. Other chapters describe how the traditional view is being extended by new findings. The writing is in a straightforward and conversational style.

D. HESTENES, *How the Brain Works. . . The Next Great Scientific Revolution*. This article is a summary and overview of the first truly coherent mathematical theory of learning, memory, and behavior consistent with experimental data. Written from the point of view of a theoretical physicist, the reference is highly recommended.

EXERCISES

1. Starting with the shunting STM equation, show that it simplifies to the additive STM equation.

2. For the system in figure 2.16, write out the additive STM and passive decay LTM equations.

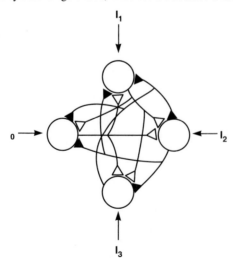

Figure 2.16 A four-neuron network for exercises 2 and 3. The open synapses are excitatory; the dark synapses are inhibitory.

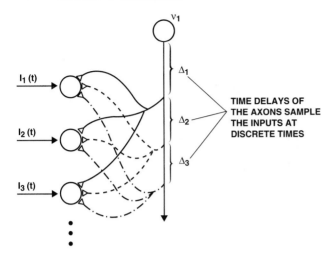

TIME DELAYS OF
THE AXONS SAMPLE
THE INPUTS AT
DISCRETE TIMES

Figure 3.5   An avalanche neural network with a single command cell. An avalanche neural network can learn a time-varying input pattern. Time delays on the command axon sample the input at selected times and store it on discrete synapse sets, with each set acting as an outstar. Thus, a single command neuron successively activates the outstars.

Sending a read-out signal from the command neuron recalls a complete space-time pattern without interruption. The read-out produces a STM pattern across the input neurons proportional to the original pattern.

Variations of avalanche architectures are readily constructed. Figure 3.6 shows an avalanche with many command neurons controlled by a single higher-level command neuron. This NN has a command neuron for each pattern.

Avalanches of avalanches allow for interrupting the learning and recalling. These NNs introduce inhibitory signals to the command cells. The operation of these NNs, however, follows directly without new insights and thus are not discussed.

Estimate the memory capacity of neuron group organized as avalanches. Assume N_s (sensor) neurons in the input layer. Assume each input pattern has a command neuron. Then, the number of neurons is $N_s + N_c$, where N_c is the number of patterns memorized.

Using avalanches, the memory capacity gives neuron populations consistent with the human brain.

For example, assume most of the patterns we learn have to do with vision (normally the dominant sense organ). About 10^6 (1000×1000) pixels are in each pattern impressed on the visual cortex. So, $N_s = 10^6$. For an upper bound, assume we memorize one pattern a second for 100 years. The number of seconds is about 3.15×10^9. So, $N_c = 3.15 \times 10^9$. Thus, the number of neurons in an avalanche capable for the task is less than 3.2×10^9. The number of neurons in the human brain is at least 10^{12}. Thus, the avalanche model is consistent.

Unquestionably, however, the structures for human memory are more complex than suggested above. These are estimates to be taken figuratively because the above model assumes large fan-outs and playback is uninterrupted once started. Nevertheless, the argument suggests the avalanche model is consistent with the massive storage capacity of biological systems.

Having described a class of elementary NNs capable of spatiotemporal pattern learning, we will modify such NNs according to the application in later chapters.

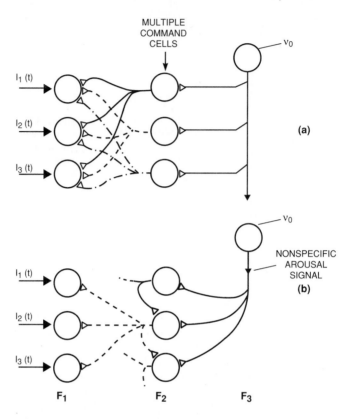

Figure 3.6   Avalanches with several command cells controlled by a single cell.
(a) A single command neuron v_0 controls other neurons that in turn sequentially
activate outstars for sampling and storing a time-varying input pattern. Thus,
different command neurons can sample the same outstar. (b) A single command
neuron v_0 in layer F_3 prepares a neural network for activation by a learning
signal. The learning signal activates neurons in layer F_2 sequentially by lateral
signals. These neurons in turn activate outstars in layer F_1. Thus, a general
arousal stimulus caused by a context prepares the outstars for learning.

3.3 INSTARS

An <u>instar</u> is a NN for recognizing spatial patterns. As with outstars, the name comes from
the geometry, shown in figure 3.7.

The mathematics of instars is like that of outstars. The differential equations for the
input neurons are

$$\dot{x}_i = -Ax_i + I_i(t), \ \forall i, \tag{3.15}$$

and for the output neuron,

$$\left.\begin{aligned}
\dot{x}_k &= -Ax_k + \sum_i S_{ik} Z_{ik}, \ \forall i, k, \\
\dot{Z}_{ik} &= -BZ_{ik} + S_{ik}[x_k]^+, \ \forall i, k.
\end{aligned}\right\} \tag{3.16}$$

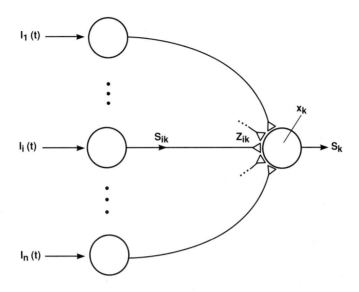

Figure 3.7   The instar neural network. This neural network learns and recognizes an input pattern. To learn, an input pattern is applied, causing signals to the center neuron. Activating the center neuron causes the long-term memory trace to go to a steady state proportional to the inputs. To recognize, another input turns on the center neuron if it is like the long-term memory trace. (Figure 3.8 shows more detail.)

To solve the differential equations, make assumptions about the coefficients and consider the steady state. As in the outstar, treat learning and recognizing separately.

1. Learning. Let reflectance coefficients represent the input pattern. That is,

$$I_i(t) = \theta_i I(t), \ \forall i. \tag{3.17}$$

Then, the steady-state STM of the input neurons is proportional to the reflectance coefficients, or

$$x_i \propto \theta_i, \ \forall i.$$

Activating the input neurons produces axon signals of the form

$$S_{ik}(t) = s_{ik} f[x_i(t - \tau_{ik}) - \Gamma_i], \ \forall i, k.$$

After relaxation $(t \gg 1/A)$, the signals are proportional to the input pattern. Assuming $x_i > \Gamma_i$,

$$S_{ik} \propto x_i \propto \theta_i, \ \forall i.$$

Let

$$S_{ik} = \mu\theta_i, \ \forall i, k, \tag{3.18}$$

where μ is a proportionality constant.

For convenience, write the LTM equations in (3.16) in matrix notation. Let,

$$
\begin{bmatrix} \dot{Z}_{1k} \\ \cdot \\ \cdot \\ \cdot \\ \dot{Z}_{Nk} \end{bmatrix} = -B \begin{bmatrix} Z_{1k} \\ \cdot \\ \cdot \\ \cdot \\ Z_{Nk} \end{bmatrix} + \begin{bmatrix} S_{1k} \\ \cdot \\ \cdot \\ \cdot \\ S_{Nk} \end{bmatrix} [x_k]^+, \ \forall k. \tag{3.19}
$$

By (3.18),

$$
\dot{\mathbf{Z}}_k = -B\mathbf{Z}_k + \mu\theta[x_k]^+, \ \forall k, \tag{3.20}
$$

where θ is the vector of reflectance coefficients.

As $t \to \infty$, $\mathbf{Z}_k$ relaxes to

$$
\mathbf{Z}_i(t) = \frac{\mu[x_k]^+}{B} N(t)\theta, \ \forall i, k. \tag{3.21}
$$

Or, if $x_k > 0$,

$$
\mathbf{Z}_k \propto \theta, \ \forall k. \tag{3.22}
$$

In words, the steady-state LTM vector is proportional to the input pattern expressed as a reflectance coefficient vector. That is, the NN learns the pattern and stores it in the LTM trace, as in outstar training.

When the instar learns more than one input pattern, the vector, $\mathbf{Z}_k$, asymptotically aligns itself with a weighted average of the reflectance vectors. This result is known as the instar code development theorem, proved by repeatedly solving (3.15) and (3.16) over discrete time intervals.

Thus, the LTM trace for M input patterns is

$$
\mathbf{Z}_k \propto f_1\theta_1 + f_2\theta_2 + \cdots + f_M\theta_M, \ \forall k, \tag{3.23}
$$

where f_i = fraction of time θ_i is present.

2. Recognition. Instar recognition is by comparing an input pattern to the stored LTM vector. Assume a new input pattern, P. The STM of an output neuron is

$$
\dot{x}_k = -Ax_k + \sum_i S_{ik} Z_{ik}, \ \forall k,
$$

where S_{ik} is proportional to the input pattern and Z_{ik} is proportional to the stored pattern (Note: $S_{ik} Z_{ik}$ can be written as a matrix dot product of $\mathbf{Z}_k$ and θ_k.)

Then, the input pattern, P, belongs to the pattern class represented by $\mathbf{Z}_k$ if it causes the output neuron to exceed threshold. As shown in figure 3.8, the output neuron fires if $x_k > \tau_k$, thus "recognizing the pattern."

In summary, instar and outstar NNs are dual to one another. When drawn in their symmetric forms, they differ only in the signal direction.

An outstar can recall but cannot recognize a pattern, while an instar can recognize but cannot recall. That is, the outstar is blind; the instar is dumb.

These two elementary NNs offer a general architecture for solving many signal processing problems. Later chapters give examples.

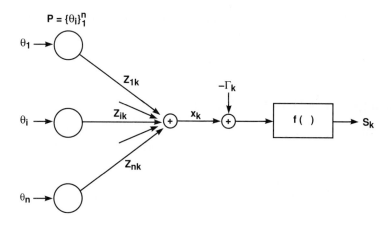

Figure 3.8   Recognition of a pattern by an instar neural network. An unknown input pattern is applied to an instar. The inputs cause signal S_i along the axon to a center neuron. The signal is multiplied by the long-term memory, summed, and compared with a threshold. If the center neuron fires, the input pattern is recognized as belonging to the pattern class represented by the long-term memory trace.

3.4 MULTIPLE INSTARS

Multiple instars can classify spatial input patterns. For example, figure 3.9 shows three instars that can classify a pattern to one of three classes. Each instar works as described in the preceding section. Select the thresholds to define the output classes.

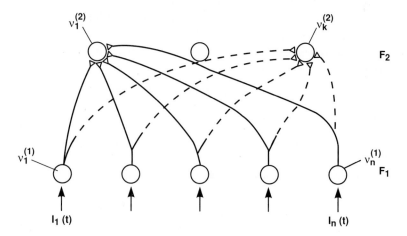

Figure 3.9   Multiple instars can classify an input pattern into one of k classes. Input neurons are in layer F_1 and the center neuron of the instars are in layer F_2. The long-term memory trace of each F_2 neuron represents a pattern class. When inputs are applied to F_1, one or more neurons in F_2 are activated showing that the input belongs to the corresponding pattern(s).

More complex NNs are built up from instars and outstars. ARTs (see section 4.2) are multiple instars and outstars designed to recall, recognize, and compare patterns. These complex NNs also do other processing tasks. Perceptrons (see section 4.4) are multiple instars, classifying inputs according to decision regions defined by training.

3.5 SIMPLE LATERAL INTERACTIONS

All NNs discussed up to this point are systems with only feedforward or feedback. That is, no connections occur among neurons lying in the same layer. This section considers simple lateral connections in a layer. Connections of this kind give a NN that is sensitive to two-dimensional shapes.

Assume a layer of interacting neurons with an input pattern. The STM trace is

$$\dot{x}_i = -\alpha_i x_i + \sum_{l \neq i}^{N} S_{li} Z_{li} - \sum_{k \neq i, l}^{N} C_{ki} + I_i, \; \forall i. \tag{3.24}$$

Assume lateral inhibition and no lateral excitations. Then,

$$\dot{x}_i = -\alpha_i x_i - \sum_{k \neq i}^{N} C_{ki} + I_i, \; \forall i.$$

Assume piecewise linear excitation for C_{ki}. Then,

$$\dot{x}_i = -\alpha_i x_i - \sum_{k \neq i}^{N} c_{ki} [x_k(t - \tau_{ki}) - \Gamma_{ki}]^+ + I_i, \; \forall i.$$

Assume negligible delay times (neurons close together). Then,

$$\dot{x}_i = -\alpha_i x_i - \sum_{k \neq i}^{N} c_{ki} [x_k(t) - \Gamma_{ki}]^+ + I_i, \; \forall i.$$

For convenience, define the excitation, e_i, of a neuron when no inhibition is present. That is, when $c_{ki} = 0$. Then,

$$\dot{e}_i = -\alpha_i e_i + I_i(t), \; \forall i.$$

Subtracting gives

$$(\dot{x}_i - \dot{e}_i) = -\alpha_i (x_i - e_i) - \sum_{k \neq i}^{N} c_{ki} [x_k(t) - \Gamma_{ki}]^+, \; \forall i.$$

Assume a constant steady state and a constant constant. Then,

$$x_i = [e_i - \sum_{k \neq i}^{N} c_{ki} [x_k - \Gamma_{ki}]^+]^+, \; \forall i. \tag{3.25}$$

This is the Hartline–Ratliff equation. Hartline, Ratliff, and others modeled the eye response of the horse-crab Limulus by (3.25) [66].

To illustrate lateral inhibitory effects with the Hartline–Ratliff equation, consider neurons in a two- dimensional triangular pattern with symmetrical inhibitory coefficients, shown in figure 3.10. Each neuron is surrounded by six adjacent neurons. Consider illuminating the array with a simple dark and light pattern. Let a pattern be defined by two straight lines at an angle, shown in figure 3.11.

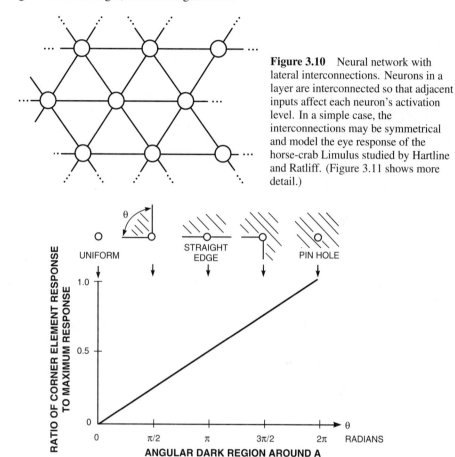

Figure 3.10   Neural network with lateral interconnections. Neurons in a layer are interconnected so that adjacent inputs affect each neuron's activation level. In a simple case, the interconnections may be symmetrical and model the eye response of the horse-crab Limulus studied by Hartline and Ratliff. (Figure 3.11 shows more detail.)

Figure 3.11   Response of a neuron that measures the angle of a corner. The eye of Limulus consists of about 1000 visual elements, called ommatidia, in an interconnected network. When an element is illuminated, it inhibits surrounding elements. The degree of inhibition measures the angle between lines in a dark-light pattern. When the element is uniformly illuminated, the response is 0, corresponding to a uniform input. When partially illuminated, the response increases and is maximum for a pinhole pattern. (Figure 3.12 shows more detail.)

By (3.25), the response of a neuron, x_i, near the corner measures the angle. That is, the neurons in the uniform dark and light have zero response while those near the edge in the light have responses that increase nearer the corner. Figure 3.11 shows that the response of a neuron near the corner as the angle defining the dark region varies from 0° to 360°.

To generalize, consider a pattern consisting of straight lines, shown in figure 3.12. The number of maxima gives the number of corners in the pattern. Moreover, because of the architecture, the number of maxima is independent of size, rotations, and translations.

Select a threshold for responses only on the corners. Thus, the architecture leads to a NN for recognizing polygons, shown in figure 3.13.

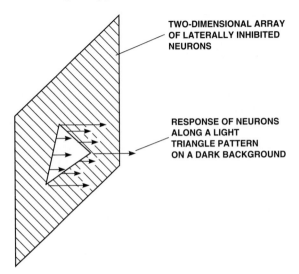

TWO-DIMENSIONAL ARRAY OF LATERALLY INHIBITED NEURONS

RESPONSE OF NEURONS ALONG A LIGHT TRIANGLE PATTERN ON A DARK BACKGROUND

Figure 3.12 Response of neurons to a triangular shape. By laterally interconnecting neurons in a layer, the response to, say, a triangular pattern is maximum at the corners. (Figure 3.13 shows more detail.)

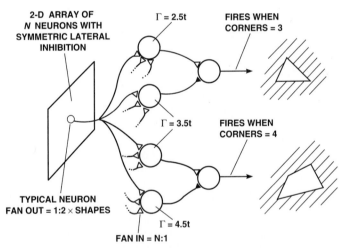

2-D ARRAY OF *N* NEURONS WITH SYMMETRIC LATERAL INHIBITION

$\Gamma = 2.5t$

FIRES WHEN CORNERS = 3

$\Gamma = 3.5t$

FIRES WHEN CORNERS = 4

TYPICAL NEURON FAN OUT = 1:2 × SHAPES

$\Gamma = 4.5t$

FAN IN = N:1

t = THRESHOLD FOR DETECTING A CORNER RESPONSE
Γ = THRESHOLD FOR COUNTING RESPONSES (Corners)

Figure 3.13 A neural network for detecting shapes regardless of size, orientation, and location. Each neuron in a neural network with lateral connects is part of an instar. By selecting the threshold, the instar can recognize geometric patterns consisting of straight lines. It follows that the number of maxima gives the number of corners in the pattern regardless of its size, location, and orientation.

(the Circadian pacemaker) discussed in the text. The idea of slow chemical activity for timing leads to an important NN module. For example, it enables modeling sleep and nocturnal activities. Moreover, from an applications viewpoint, a gated dipole can be the master oscillator of a system.

EXERCISES

1. Some characteristics of the human auditory system are

   a. Frequency Range: 20–20,000 Hz
   b. Relative discrimination of different tones: 1800 "just noticeable differences" at 60 dB

   Assume the system works by sampling the output of a bank of 1800 frequency filters. Assume the sampling rate is $2\times$ the maximum frequency.

   a. Estimate the number of neurons needed to memorize Beethoven's 9th Symphony (time = 64 minutes), assuming an avalanche-type neural network.
   b. What fan-out is needed from each command neuron to the sensor array neurons?
   c. Sketch the avalanche structure.

2. Consider a two-input outstar shown in figure 3.17:

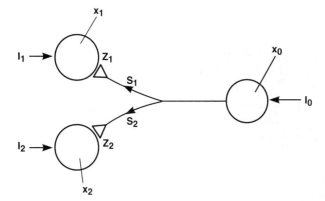

Figure 3.17   Neural network for exercise 2.

   a. Write the Additive STM and Passive Decay LTM equations for this system.
   b. Simplify the equations by assuming negligible delay times and thresholds.
   c. Assume the following inputs for I_1 and I_2:

$$I_1 = \begin{cases} \frac{1}{2}\sin \omega t & 0 \le t < 2 \\ \frac{1}{4}\sin \omega t & 2 \le t < 3 \\ 0, & 3 \le t \end{cases}$$

$$I_2 = \begin{cases} \frac{1}{2}\sin \omega t & 0 \le t < 2 \\ \frac{3}{4}\sin \omega t & 2 \le t < 3 \\ 0, & 3 \le t \end{cases}$$

   What is the steady-state value of the LTM trace for $t > 3$?

3. Consider the following system shown in figure 3.18:

   a. Write the Additive STM and Passive Decay LTM equations for this system assuming negligible delay times and thresholds.
   b. Assume a piecewise linear function for S_1 and S_2, all coefficients = unity magnitude, $x_1, x_2 > 0$, and $I_1 > I_2$. What is the steady-state value for the STM when $I_0 = 0$?

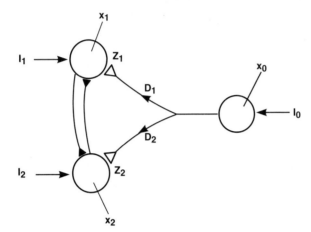

Figure 3.18   Neural network for exercise 3.

4. Consider simulating two characteristics of a Rana Catesbeiana (frog).

   a. An insect crossing the field of view (FOV) causes the tongue to catch it.
   b. A large shadow crossing the FOV causes the frog to jump.

   These reflexes are automatic without involving higher brain centers. Using the elementary neural network modules developed to date, design a neural network implementing these characteristics.

5. Consider a shunting STM equation,

$$\dot{x}_i = -Ax_i + (B - x_i)I_i(t), \; \forall i.$$

   a. Find the steady-state response.
   b. Given initial value $x_i(0)$, solve for $x_i(t)$ for time $t > 0$.
   c. How does the rate of $x_i(t)$ approaching its steady state depend on I_i?

4

Complex Networks

The preceding chapter derived simple NN modules and illustrated standard mathematical techniques. This chapter describes complex networks and their properties starting with a general class of NNs. The chapter discusses the major design problems, such as noise-saturation and stability-plasticity tradeoffs.

4.1 COOPERATIVE-COMPETITIVE SYSTEMS

Cooperative-competitive (CC) NNs are complex systems of interconnected excitatory and inhibitory neurons.

CC NNs are difficult to analyze because of the nonlinear signal function (see chapter 2). This section considers topics about CC NNs. The approach considers the simplest CC systems first and then builds up to more complex systems. Examples illustrate the mechanisms responsible for network properties.

The simple NNs of chapter 3 ignored two important issues: noise and saturation. Noise is important because many biological NNs operate near the quantum limit, for example, vision. Saturation is important because neurons have finite operating ranges. Saturation means larger signals do not cause larger responses.

A NN may need a wide dynamic range between the noise floor and a saturation limit because of wide fluctuations in signal levels.

The dynamic range issue in NN theory is called the noise-saturation dilemma, and is well known to designers of electronic circuits. The noise-saturation dilemma is as follows.

If the NN is sensitive to large inputs, how does it distinguish small inputs from internal noise? If the NN is sensitive to small inputs, how does it remain responsive to large inputs? The following sections analyze the noise-saturation dilemma starting with simple CC systems.

1. Interacting Neurons and Groups of NNs. Assume the shunting STM model that models axon membrane characteristics. As shown in chapter 2, the activation is

$$\dot{x}_i = -A_i x_i + (B_i - x_i)[\sum_j C_{ji} f(x_j) Z_{ji}^{(+)} + I_i]$$
$$- (x_i + D_i)[\sum_k E_{ki} g(x_k) Z_{ki}^{(-)} + J_i], \forall i. \tag{4.1}$$

Note that A_i, B_i, C_{ji}, D_i, and E_{ji} are positive. By considering the sign of $\dot{x}_i$, the steady-state $\bar{x}_i$ is between $-D_i$ and B_i.

Equation (4.1) describes interacting neurons or interacting groups of neurons. When interpreted as interacting neurons, the coefficients are axon membrane parameters. When interpreted as interacting groups, B_i is the excitable neurons in the NN denoted by v_i. Of this number, x_i are excited and B_i-x_i are unexcited. ($x_i < 0$ means the NN is hyperpolarized, needing excitation first to $x_i = 0$ and then to $x_i > 0$.)

2. Simplest Network with Automatic Gain Control. Apply (4.1) to the system shown in figure 4.1. This system is an on-center/off-surround (ON CTR/OFF SUR) feedforward NN. As shown, an input to a neuron tends to turn on the neuron while tending to turn off adjacent neurons. This system has no interactions among the neurons.

Writing $J_i = \sum_{k \neq i} I_k$, (4.1) simplifies to

$$\dot{x}_i = -A x_i + (B - x_i) I_i - (x_i + D) \sum_{k \neq i} I_k, \forall i. \tag{4.2}$$

Rearranging the terms of (4.2) gives

$$\dot{x}_i = -A x_i + (B I_i - D \sum_{k \neq i} I_k) - x_i (I_i + \sum_{k \neq i} I_k), \forall i.$$

Setting $\dot{x}_i = 0$ and solving for the steady state gives

$$\bar{x}_i = \frac{B I_i - D \sum_{k \neq i} I_k}{A + I_i + \sum_{k \neq i} I_k}, \forall i. \tag{4.3}$$

Assume no lateral interactions, that is $\sum_{k \neq i} I_k = 0$. Then

$$\bar{x}_i = \frac{B I_i}{A + I_i} \xrightarrow{I_i \to \infty} B. \tag{4.4}$$

For this NN, each $x_i(t)$ saturates at B for large inputs, regardless of the input pattern. A system needs lateral interactions to avoid saturation.

Consider a system with lateral interaction terms. Rewrite (4.3) as

$$\bar{x}_i = \frac{B I_i - D(I - I_i)}{A + I}, \forall i, \tag{4.5}$$

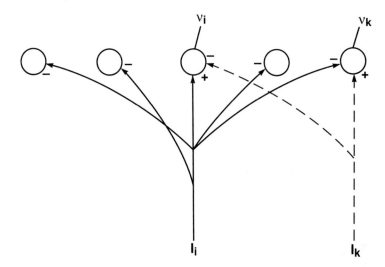

Figure 4.1   An on-center/off-surround feedforward neural network with automatic gain control. Input I_i excites neuron v_i while inhibiting the other neurons. A second input I_k excites neuron v_k and inhibits v_i. The system has automatic gain control. That is, the steady-state responses remain proportional to large inputs.

where

$$I = I_i + \sum_{k \neq i} I_k, \ \forall i. \tag{4.6}$$

With lateral interactions, the steady state has the form

$$\bar{x}_i = \frac{(B+D)I}{A+I}(\theta_i - \frac{D}{B+D}), \ \forall i, \tag{4.7}$$

where $\theta_i = I_i/I$ are the reflectance coefficients (see chapter 3).

The first term, $(B+D)I/A+I$, gives information about the background by I. The second term, $(\theta_i - D/(B+D))$, gives information about the pattern by θ_i. The term $D/(B+D)$ is called the adaptation level.

With lateral interactions, the steady-state response still gives pattern information for large inputs. That is,

$$\bar{x}_i \xrightarrow{I \to \infty} (B+D)(\theta_i - \frac{D}{B+D}), \ \forall i. \tag{4.8}$$

Thus, in electrical engineering terminology, the system has automatic gain control.

3. Noise Suppression. Equation (4.7) shows θ_i must exceed $D/(B+D)$ to excite the NN. Assume N inputs, $I_1, I_2, \ldots, I_N$. Setting the adaptation level to $1/N$ gives

$$\bar{x}_i = \frac{(B+D)I}{A+I}(\theta_i - \frac{1}{N}), \ \forall i. \tag{4.9}$$

This system has noise suppression in its simplest form. That is, for a uniform (noisy) input, $(\theta_i = 1/N)$, $\bar{x}_i = 0$, $\forall i$.

4. Pattern Matching. The noise suppression brings about pattern matching in the following sense. Assume each input I_i is the sum of two inputs J_i and K_i. That is, $I_i = J_i + K_i$, $\forall i$, corresponding to patterns $J = (J_1, \ldots, J_N)$ and $K = (K_1, \ldots, K_N)$.

The NN compares patterns J and K as follows. If J and K are mismatched, their peaks and troughs tend to produce a uniform pattern. Thus, the neurons will be inhibited and their steady-state response tends to zero. (The next section develops this property.)

If the two patterns are matched, they reinforce each other. For perfect matching, that is, $J_i = \alpha K_i$, the steady-state response is

$$\bar{x}_i = \frac{[B + D(1+\alpha)\bar{K}]}{[A + (1+\alpha)\bar{K}]}(\theta_i - \frac{1}{N}), \forall i, \tag{4.10}$$

where $\bar{K} = \sum_i K_i$. Thus, matching J and K amplifies the steady-state response without changing the pattern θ_i.

The preceding ON CTR/OFF SUR NN explains some empirical results.

The Weber–Fechner law (W–F law) is a well-known psychophysics result found in variety of sensory phenomena. The W–F law says that over a broad range of input values

$$\frac{\Delta I}{I} = \text{constant}, \tag{4.11}$$

where ΔI is the "just noticeable" input difference compared with a background input I. (See table 1.5 for vision, hearing, and touch thresholds in human beings.)

NN considerations can derive the W–F law. Starting with (4.7), let

$$I' = I + \Delta I.$$

Substituting gives

$$\bar{x}_i' = \frac{(B + D)(I + \Delta I)}{A + I + \Delta I}(\theta_i - \frac{D}{B+D}).$$

Assume $A + I \gg \Delta I$. Then,

$$\frac{\bar{x}_i'}{\bar{x}_i} = 1 + \frac{\Delta I}{I},$$

or

$$\frac{\Delta \bar{x}_i}{\bar{x}_i} = \frac{\Delta I}{I}.$$

Interpreting this result, if $\Delta \bar{x}_i/\bar{x}_i$ is the "just noticeable" difference in the NN response, $\Delta I/I = $ constant as observed.

Another empirical result, about brightness, can also be explained. Let $\bar{X}$ be the total steady-state activity. That is,

$$\bar{X} = \sum_i \bar{x}_i. \tag{4.12}$$

By (4.7)

$$\bar{X} = \frac{(B+D)I}{A+I}(1 - N\frac{D}{B+D}).\tag{4.13}$$

Thus, if $D/(B+D) = 1/N$, $\bar{X} = 0$. That is, for a network receiving a fixed illuminance, if one part is made brighter (increasing $\bar{x}_i$), the other part is darker (decreasing $\bar{x}_i$). This property explains the brightness contrast illustrated in figure 4.2.

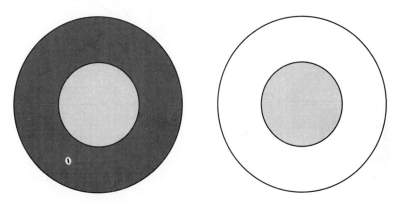

Figure 4.2   Example of brightness contrast. For an on-center/off-surround neural network with fixed input, if responses of one part increase, the responses of the remaining part decrease. To illustrate, the central area on the right looks darker than the identical central area on the left because the surround on the right is lighter than the surround on the left.

5. Noise Suppression and Contrast Improvement.   Lateral interactions between inputs and responses produce other NN properties. Figure 4.3 shows a simple system with feedback. Equation (4.14) describes the system.

$$\dot{x}_i = -A_i x_i + (B_i - x_i)[f(x_i) + I_i] - x_i[\sum_{k \neq i} f(x_k) + J_i], \forall i \tag{4.14}$$

where

$$0 < \bar{x}_i < B.$$

Assume I_i and J_i act before $t = 0$ to establish an initial activation pattern, $x_1(0), \ldots, x_N(0)$.

After removing the inputs, the response for $t > 0$ is

$$\dot{x}_i = -A_i x_i + (B_i - x_i)f(x_i) - x_i \sum_{k \neq i} f(x_k), \forall i. \tag{4.15}$$

The kind of the feedback signal function, $f(\ )$, affects the steady-state responses. Figure 4.4 shows the initial activation pattern at the top. The left column shows possible functions for $f(x_i)$, while the middle column shows the steady-state responses.

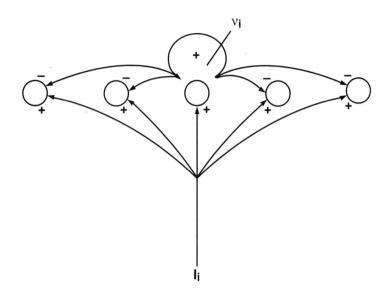

Figure 4.3   An on-center/off-surround neural network with feedback. The lateral feedback interactions among the neurons produce noise suppression and contrast enhancement.

When $f(x_i)$ is slower than linear, noise is amplified and the response is uniform, that is, the network experiences seizure. When $f(x_i)$ is linear, the pattern is unchanged and the systems amplifies noise and signal equally. When $f(x_i)$ is faster than linear, noise is suppressed and the maximum is a unique winner-takes-all.

Combining these results, noise is suppressed and the signal is amplified when $f(x_i)$ is sigmoidal. The quenching threshold, QT, defines noise and signal. That is, signal is $x_i \geq QT$; noise is $x_i < QT$.

For this simple system, the quenching threshold can be calculated and is

$$QT = \frac{x_l}{x_u - \frac{A}{S}}, \tag{4.16}$$

where figure 4.4 defines x_l, x_u, and S.

6. Temporal Stability and the Stability-Plasticity Dilemma. NN theory has two stability issues. First, is the temporal stability, well known from conventional systems theory. Stability in this sense has to do with the asymptotic behavior at large times.

Few general temporal stability conditions are known for the STM and LTM state equations. One well-known result is the Cohen–Grossberg theorem for STM temporal stability in the sense of Lyapunov.

Lyapunov's approach is to associate an energy function, $V(t)$ (the Lyapunov function) with the system. If this function decreases as time increases, energy is leaving the system so the system relaxes to zero. In practice, however, finding a Lyapunov function for the system may be difficult.

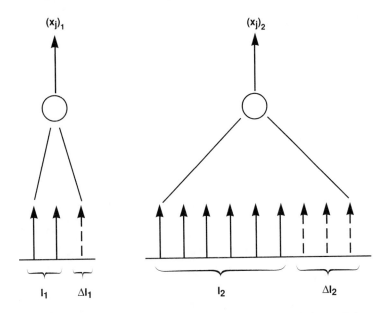

Figure 4.7   The Weber–Fechner law is that the response to a change in input, ΔI, depends on the relative change $\Delta I / I$. The ART-1 algorithm gives the same response if $\Delta I_1 / I_1 = \Delta I_2 / I_2$, as shown.

If a minimum δx_j is just noticeable, say $\delta x_j = (\Delta x_j)_{threshold}$, (4.38) gives

$$x_j \approx \frac{(\Delta x_j)_{threshold}}{\text{constant}}, \; \forall j.$$

Thus,

$$x_j \approx \text{constant} \Rightarrow |I|\hat{Z}_{ij} = \text{constant}.$$

That is, for a W–F law response, increasing the active F_1 nodes decreases the magnitude of Z_{ij} (the LTM trace).

To build this relationship in E_{ij}, assume competition among the Z_{ij} terms for synaptic sites. Let

$$E_{ij} = h(x_i) + \frac{1}{L}\sum_{k \neq i} h(x_k), \; \forall i, j \tag{4.39}$$

and

$$k_1 = KL. \tag{4.40}$$

Substituting in (4.35) gives

$$\dot{Z}_{ij} = Kf(x_j)[(1 - Z_{ij})Lh(x_i) - Z_{ij}\sum_{k \neq i} h(x_k)]. \tag{4.41}$$

The size of Z_{ij} depends on the number of active nodes. That is,

$$\bar{Z}_{ij} = \frac{Lh(x_i)}{Lh(x_i) + \sum_{k \neq i} h(x_k)} \propto \frac{1}{|\mathcal{X}|},$$

where $|\mathcal{X}|$ is the active F_1 nodes and L is the relative strength of bottom-up competition among the LTM traces. L small (near one) implies stronger LTM competition.

Figure 4.8 illustrates the response to subsets and supersets. When input $I^{(1)}$ is impressed, the F_2 response is largest at v_1, because $(Z_{ij})_1 > (Z_{ij})_2$. When input $I^{(2)}$ is impressed, containing $I^{(1)}$, the response is largest at v_2. In this way ART-1 distinguishes a set and a superset.

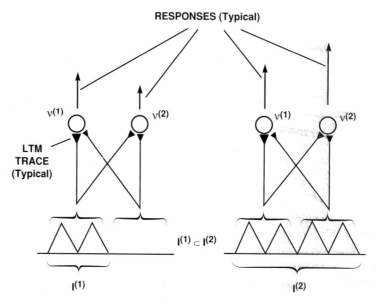

RESPONSES (Typical)

$\nu(1)$ $\nu(2)$

LTM
TRACE
(Typical)

$I^{(1)} \subset I^{(2)}$

$I^{(1)}$

$\nu(1)$ $\nu(2)$

$I^{(2)}$

Figure 4.8 ART-1 contains the Weber–Fechner law by making the long-term memory traces inversely proportional to the activated F_1 neurons. Then, ART-1 can distinguish a subset $I^{(1)}$ from a superset $I^{(2)}$, as shown.

Further simplify by assuming

$$\left.\begin{array}{l} f(x_j) = 1, \quad x_j \text{ ON}, \\ h(x_k) = 1, \quad x_k \text{ ON}. \end{array}\right\} \tag{4.42}$$

Then

$$\dot{Z}_{ij} = \left\{ \begin{array}{ll} K[(1 - Z_{ij}L - Z_{ij}(|\mathcal{X}| - 1), & v_i, v_j \text{ ON}, \\ -K|\mathcal{X}|Z_{ij}, & v_i \text{ OFF}, v_j \text{ ON}, \\ 0, & v_j \text{ OFF}. \end{array} \right. \tag{4.43}$$

Assume fast learning. That is, by (4.43) the steady-state LTM is

$$\bar{Z}_{ij} = \left\{ \begin{array}{ll} \frac{L}{L-1+|\mathcal{X}|}, & v_i, v_j \text{ ON}, \\ 0, & v_i \text{ OFF}, v_j \text{ ON}. \end{array} \right. \tag{4.44}$$

Turning next to the $F_2 \rightarrow F_1$ (top-down) LTM trace, assume a gated dipole model, that is

$$\dot{Z}_{ji} = k_2 f(x_j)[-E_{ij}Z_{ij} + h(x_i)], \; \forall i, j. \tag{4.45}$$

Assume $E_{ij} = 1$, giving

$$\dot{Z}_{ji} = f(x_j)[-Z_{ij} + h(x_i)].$$

Assume

$$\left. \begin{array}{ll} f(x_j) = 1, & x_j \text{ ON,} \\ h(x_i) = 1, & x_k \text{ ON,} \end{array} \right\} \tag{4.46}$$

to give

$$\dot{Z}_{ji} = \begin{cases} -Z_{ji} + 1, & v_i, v_j \text{ ON,} \\ -Z_{ji}, & v_i \text{ OFF, } v_j \text{ ON,} \\ 0, & v_j \text{ OFF.} \end{cases} \tag{4.47}$$

Assuming fast learning gives

$$\bar{Z}_{ji} = \begin{cases} 1, & v_i, v_j \text{ ON,} \\ 0, & v_i \text{ OFF, } v_j \text{ ON.} \end{cases} \tag{4.48}$$

When a mismatch happens on F_1, a more uniform activity pattern appears. This uniformity leads to a decrease in the active nodes, that is, $|\mathcal{X}|$ decreases. When F_2 is not active, $|\mathcal{X}| = |I|$. When F_2 is active and mismatched, $|\mathcal{X}| < |I|$.

Define ρ (the vigilance) so that if

$$\frac{|\mathcal{X}|}{|\mathcal{I}|} < \rho, \, 0 < \rho \le 1, \tag{4.49}$$

reset occurs.

Assume reset inhibits the currently active F_2 node for a prolonged time. Define $f(x_j)$ so that

$$f(x_j) = \begin{cases} 1, & \text{if } T_j = \max\{T_k | k \epsilon \mathcal{J}\}, \\ 0, & \text{otherwise.} \end{cases}$$

where $\mathcal{J}$ is the set of indices of F_2 nodes that may be activated.

At first,

$$\mathcal{J} = \{M + 1, M + 2, \ldots, N\}. \tag{4.50}$$

Assume a rule for matching input and LTM traces, called the 2/3 Rule (defined below). The system needs this rule because readout of V^J (outstar) may activate some F_1 nodes not previously activated by the input I alone. This activation would result in preventing the input from being encoded in the F_2 LTM. Moreover, a single node in F_2 may code disjoint input patterns, despite the fact the two patterns shared no features.

The 2/3 rule controls which v_i in F_1 remains active. Let $\mathcal{I}$ be the indice set receiving positive inputs. That is,

$$\mathcal{I} = \{1, 2, \ldots, M\}. \tag{4.51}$$

Let V^J be the indices of F_1 that are ON when v_J is ON.

Example: For the situation in figure 4.9, $\mathcal{I} = \{1, 2, 4, 5\}$ and $v_J = \{1, 3, 5\}$. If $\mathcal{X}$ is the indice set of F_1 that are ON, the 2/3 rule is

$$\mathcal{X} = \begin{cases} \mathcal{I}, & \text{if } F_2 \text{ OFF,} \\ \mathcal{I} \cap V^{(J)}, & \text{if } v_j \in F_2 \text{ ON.} \end{cases} \tag{4.52}$$

For the figure 4.9 example, $\mathcal{X} = \{1, 5\}$.

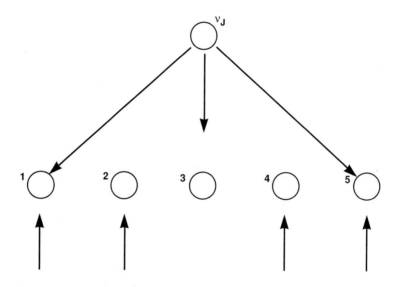

Figure 4.9   Example of ART-1. An ART-1 with five F_1 nodes has external inputs to v_1, v_2, v_3, v_4 and v_5. A F_2 node activates and produces more inputs to nodes $v_1, v_3,$ and v_5 by the $F_2 \rightarrow F_1$ long-term memory trace.

Summarizing ART-1, the algorithm is as follows. For a binary pattern I, with components I_i,

$$I_i = \begin{cases} 1, & \text{if } i \epsilon \mathcal{I}, \\ 0, & \text{otherwise.} \end{cases} \tag{4.53}$$

The bottom-up activation is

$$T_j = D_2 \sum_{i \in X} Z_{ij}, \ \forall j. \tag{4.54}$$

The F_2 node turned-on is

$$f(x_j) = \begin{cases} 1, & \text{if } T_j = \max\{T_k | k \epsilon \mathcal{J}\}, \\ 0, & \text{otherwise,} \end{cases}$$

where $\mathcal{J}$ are the indices that may be activated.

Apply the 2/3 rule for F_1 activation:

$$\mathcal{X} = \begin{cases} \mathcal{I}, & \text{if } F_2 \text{ OFF}, \\ \mathcal{I} \cap V^{(J)}, & \text{if } v_j \epsilon F_2 \text{ ON}. \end{cases}$$

Reset (zero-out) the current F_2 node for the duration of the input if

$$\frac{|\mathcal{X}|}{|\mathcal{I}|} < \rho, \ 0 < \rho \leq 1, \tag{4.55}$$

where ρ is given. If reset does not happen, update the LTM traces using fast learning.

$$Z_{ij} = \begin{cases} \frac{L}{L-1+|\mathcal{X}|}, & v_i, v_j \text{ ON } (i \in \mathcal{X}), \\ 0, & v_i \text{ OFF}, v_j \text{ ON } (i \in \mathcal{X}), \end{cases} \tag{4.56}$$

and

$$Z_{ji} = \begin{cases} 1, & v_i, v_j \text{ ON}, \\ 0, & v_i \text{ OFF}, v_j \text{ ON}. \end{cases} \tag{4.57}$$

The initial bottom-up LTM trace is

$$0 < Z_{ij}(0) < \frac{L}{L-1+M}, \tag{4.58}$$

where L and M are given.

The inequality allows direct access. That is, if v_j has learned an input, v_j is the first node chosen during search. The initial top-down LTM trace is

$$\bar{Z} = \frac{B_1 - 1}{D_1} < Z_{Ji}(0) < 1,$$

where $\max\{1, D_1\} < B_1 < 1 + D_1$.

Consider a simple example of ART-1. Figure 4.10 shows the problem, with $M = 3$, $N = 5$. Let $L = 2$. Then

$$0 < Z_{ij}(0) < \frac{L}{L-1+M} = 1/2.$$

Assume for $Z_{ij}(0)$. In matrix form for convenience,

$$[Z_{ij}(0)] = \begin{bmatrix} 1/4 & 1/8 \\ 1/4 & 1/8 \\ 1/4 & 1/8 \end{bmatrix}.$$

Let $D_1 = 1$ and $B_1 = 3/2$. The initial top-down LTM is $\bar{Z} < Z_{ji} < 1$, where

$$\bar{Z} = \frac{B_1 - 1}{D_1} = 1/2.$$

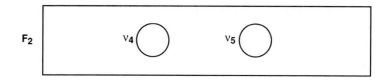

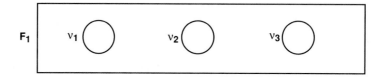

Figure 4.10 Example ART-1 neural network.

Assume

$$[Z_{ji}(0)] = \begin{bmatrix} 3/4 & 3/4 & 3/4 \\ 3/4 & 3/4 & 3/4 \end{bmatrix}.$$

Assume $I^{(1)}$ shown in figure 4.10. If v_i ON, assume $D_2 = 1$ and $h(x_i) = 1$. Then, the inputs to F_2 are

$$T_4 = \sum_i Z_{i4} = Z_{14} + Z_{24} = 1/2,$$
$$T_5 = \sum_i Z_{i5} = Z_{15} + Z_{25} = 1/4.$$

Thus, v_4 is ON and v_5 is OFF because $T_4 > T_5$. Applying the 2/3 rule,

$$\mathcal{X} = \mathcal{I} \bigcap V^{(J)} = \mathcal{I} \bigcap V^{(4)},$$

where

$$v_i \in V^{(4)} \text{ if } Z_{4i} > \bar{Z} = 1/2,$$

giving

$$\mathcal{X} = \{1, 2\} \bigcap \{1, 2, 3\} = \{1, 2\}.$$

The reset test gives

$$\frac{|\mathcal{X}|}{|\mathcal{I}|} = \frac{2}{2} = 1.$$

That is, no reset occurs. Thus, learning takes place. Fast learning gives

$$Z_{ij} = \frac{L}{L - 1 + |\mathcal{X}|} = \frac{2}{2 - 1 + 2} = 2/3, \; v_i, v_j \text{ ON,}$$
$$Z_{14} = Z_{24} = 2/3, \; Z_{34} = 0,$$
$$Z_{ji} = 1, \; v_i, v_j \text{ ON,}$$
$$Z_{41} = Z_{42} = 1, \; Z_{34} = 0.$$

After $I^{(1)}$ is applied, the bottom-up LTM traces are

$$[Z_{ij}(0)] = \begin{bmatrix} 2/3 & 1/8 \\ 2/3 & 1/8 \\ 0 & 1/8 \end{bmatrix},$$

and the top-down LTM traces are

$$[Z_{ji}(0)] = \begin{bmatrix} 1 & 1 & 0 \\ 3/4 & 3/4 & 3/4 \end{bmatrix}.$$

Continuing with $I^{(2)}$, shown in figure 4.10, after learning

$$[Z_{ij}(0)] = \begin{bmatrix} 2/3 & 0 \\ 2/3 & 2/3 \\ 0 & 2/3 \end{bmatrix},$$

and

$$[Z_{ji}(0)] = \begin{bmatrix} 1 & 1 & 0 \\ 0 & 1 & 1 \end{bmatrix}.$$

This simple system can learn only two patterns because F_2 has two nodes.

In summary, the ART-1 algorithm can learn and recognize binary patterns. In real-world applications, use processing to give the binary inputs. One extension is analog input patterns, considered next.

    2. <u>ART-2</u>. ART-2 extends ART-1. The characteristics of ART-2 are as follows.

1. ART-2 can handle binary or analog (gray-scale, continuous-valued) inputs.

2. ART-2 has the same overall structure as ART-1, that is, two layers F_1 and F_2.

3. ART-2 matches the input and LTM trace by an L_2 metric. (ART-1 matched by counting bits—the Hamming metric.) F_1 includes noise suppression and contrast improvement. Thus, the input may be noisy. (Contrast improvement is not an issue with ART-1.)

4. ART-2 normalizes the input patterns so the dynamic range may be large and considers patterns that are multiples of each other the same.

Figure 4.6 shows a flow diagram of the ART-2 algorithm. The step-by-step operation of ART-2 is as follows.

1. Present an input pattern across the bottom of F_1. The resulting STM activity in F_1 excites instar nodes on F_2. Lateral interactions in F_2 pick the maximum response and suppresses the other nodes. The surviving node on F_2 excites an outstar in F_1.

2. Apply the outstar pattern to the top of F_1, allowing a comparison between the filtered input and a LTM trace. A match reexcites the current instar on F_2, leading to increased STM activity on F_1. That is, <u>resonance</u> takes place. Resonance associates the node in F_2 with the input pattern.

3. Update the LTMs of F_1 and F_2. If a match does not happen, the comparison on F_1 leads to a more uniform input, and the F_1 STM activity decreases.

4. If the decrease is below a threshold (the vigilance), reset F_2. The reset zeros-out the current active node in F_2 by a gated dipole.

5. Reestablish the original input pattern and reexcite the instars. Choose a new F_2 maximum.

6. Compare a new outstar pattern with the filtered input.

7. Continue the sequence until matching (resonance), or until no nodes remain to be activated on F_2.

8. Reinitial the F_1 and F_2 fields before each new input pattern.

With notation from chapter 3, the equations for the ART-2 are as follows. Starting with the F_1 layer, F_1 consists of three levels shown in figure 4.11. F_1 has the following characteristics:

1. The three levels allow amplifying the input pattern in the bottom and middle levels, while suppressing noise.

2. Readout of a top-down LTM pattern, to match with the STM pattern at the top F_1 level, does not change the STM patterns of the bottom and middle layers. This decoupling

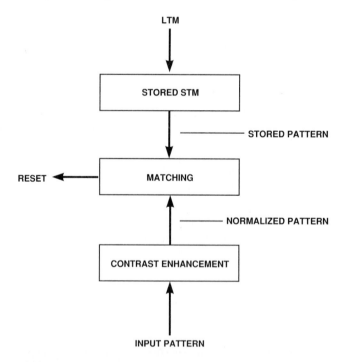

Figure 4.11   Architecture of the ART-2 F_1 layer. The F_1 layer consists of three levels, which roughly operate as follows. The bottom level filters by enhancing and normalizing the input. The long-term memory activates the top level, restoring a past pattern. The middle level compares the filtered input and a stored pattern. If mismatch occurs, the system RESETs and continues.

ensures that the LTM traces do not affect the amplifying and the noise suppression. The decoupling handles the stability-plasticity dilemma.

3. The top-down LTM trace learns the STM pattern, called the exemplar, produced at the top level of F_1. As learning takes place, the LTM trace changes. A mismatch caused by learning does not reset F_2.

Figure 4.12 shows the three F_1 levels in detail. Each input node, I_i, is associated with six nodes, labeled p_i, q_i, u_i, v_i, x_i, and w_i. The shunting STM equation describes node activation. That is,

$$\epsilon \dot{V}_i = -AV_i + (1 - BV_i)J_i^+ - (C + DV_i)J_i^-, \tag{4.59}$$

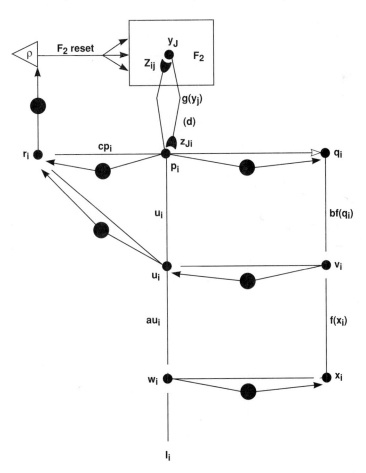

Figure 4.12   Details of the ART-2 F_1 layer. Each input I_i to F_1 has six neurons in three levels. The dark circles denote normalizing. The text gives the activation equations. (From Carpenter and Grossberg. ART-2: Self-Organization of Stable Category Recognition Codes for Analog Input Patterns in *Applied Optics*, Vol. 26. Reprinted by permission of G. Carpenter and The Optical Society of America, 1987).

where ϵ is the ratio of STM-to-LTM relaxation times, with $0 < \epsilon \ll 1$. J_i^+ is the total excitatory inputs; J_i^- is the total inhibitory inputs.

Assuming $B, C = 0$ in (4.59), the steady-state STM of a F_1 node is

$$\bar{V}_i = \frac{J_i^+}{A + DJ_i^-}. \tag{4.60}$$

Construct ART-2 by specifying equations for J_i^+ and J_i^- and by giving the connections between the nodes.

The STM equations for the top, middle, and bottom levels are

$$p_i = u_i + \sum_j g(y_j)Z_{ji}, \tag{4.61}$$

$$q_i = \frac{p_i}{e + ||p||}, \tag{4.62}$$

$$u_i = \frac{v_i}{e + ||v||}, \tag{4.63}$$

$$v_i = f(x_i) + bf(q_i), \tag{4.64}$$

$$w_i = I_i + au_i, \tag{4.65}$$

and

$$x_i = \frac{w_i}{e + ||w||}. \tag{4.66}$$

Continuing with F_2, the STM is the same as ART-1. That is, let T_j be the input from F_1.

$$T_j = \sum_i p_i Z_{ij}. \tag{4.67}$$

Assume for the F_2 STM trace, y_j, that lateral interactions causes $y_j \to 0$ for $j \neq J$, where

$$T_J = \max_j \{T_j, \ j = M + 1, \ldots, N\}. \tag{4.68}$$

Reset F_2 (by a gated dipole field in F_2), giving

$$g(y_J) = \begin{cases} d, & \text{if } T_J = \max_j\{T_j\} \text{ not previously reset,} \\ 0, & \text{otherwise.} \end{cases} \tag{4.69}$$

Thus,

$$p_i = \begin{cases} u_i, & \text{if } F_2 \text{ inactive,} \\ u_i + dZ_{Ji}, & \text{if } v_J \in F_2 \text{ is active,} \end{cases} \tag{4.70}$$

where $0 < d < 1$.

Turning to the LTM, the top-down LTM trace is

$$\dot{Z}_{ji} = g(y_j)(p_i - Z_{ji}). \tag{4.71}$$

The bottom-up LTM trace is

$$\dot{Z}_{ij} = g(y_j)(p_i - Z_{ij}). \tag{4.72}$$

Note Z_{ij}, $Z_{ji} = 0$ if $y_j = 0$. That is, for $j \neq J$.
For v_J active and v_j inactive, $j \neq J$ by (4.70). Then,

$$\dot{Z}_{ij} = d(p_i - Z_{ij}) = d(u_i + dZ_{Ji} - Z_{Ji}).$$

That is, for the top-down LTM trace

$$\dot{Z}_{Ji} = d(1 - d)(\frac{u_i}{1 - d} - Z_{Ji}). \tag{4.73}$$

Similarly, for the bottom-up LTM trace

$$\dot{Z}_{iJ} = d(1 - d)(\frac{u_i}{1 - d} - Z_{iJ}). \tag{4.74}$$

ART-2 uses a L_2 norm for measuring the degree of matching. Let

$$r_i = \frac{u_i + cp_i}{e + ||u|| + ||cp||}, \tag{4.75}$$

where $||r||$ is a L_2 norm of $r = (r_1, \ldots, r_M)$, that is,

$$||r|| = \sqrt{r_1^2 + \ldots + r_M^2}. \tag{4.76}$$

The norm, $||r||$, measures the match between the input, u_i, and stored LTM, p_i. By algebraic manipulation,

$$||r|| = \frac{1 + 2||cp||cos(u, p) + ||cp||^2}{1 + ||cp||}. \tag{4.77}$$

Write (4.77) with $Z_J = (Z_{J1}, \ldots, Z_{JM})$. That is,

$$||r|| = \frac{[(1 + c)^2 + 2(1 + c)||cdZ_J||cos(u, Z_J) + ||cdZ_J||^2]^{1/2}}{1 + [c^2 + 2c||cdZ_J||cos(u, Z_J) + ||cdZ_J||^2]^{1/2}}. \tag{4.78}$$

Figure 4.13 shows that over the range $||cdZJ|| < 1$ the norm $||r||$ is a matching parameter. The vertical coordinate gives the degree of matching. The horizontal coordinate gives the degree of learning, or sensitivity. For increased sensitivity with increased learning (larger Z_J), assume $||cdZJ|| < 1$.
By (4.73) the steady-state $\bar{Z}_{Ji} = \frac{u_i}{(1-d)}$. The constraint $||cdZ_J|| < 1$ becomes

$$\frac{cd}{1 - d} < 1. \tag{4.79}$$

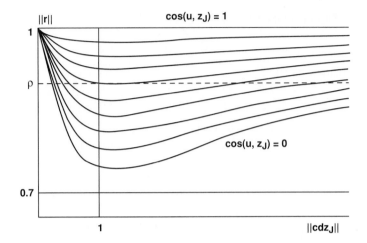

Figure 4.13 Plot of the ART-2 norm that gauges matching. $||r||$, which is a function of $\cos(u, p)$ and $||cdZ_J||$, matches the filtered input pattern, u, and a stored pattern, p. Restricting $||cdZ_J|| < 1$ shows $||r|| = 1$ for a perfect match and $||r|| = 0$ for u and p orthogonal. ART-2 is reset if $||r||$ is below the vigilance parameter ρ, which adjusts matching sensitivity. (From Carpenter and Grossberg. ART-2: Self-Organization of Stable Category Recognition Codes for Analog Input Patterns in *Applied Optics*, Vol. 26. Reprinted by permission of G. Carpenter and The Optical Society of America, 1987).

Thus, the closer $cd/(1-d)$ is to one, the more sensitive the system. The learning categories are also more stable. Thus, initial categories are the same as later categories (stability in the encoding sense).

Reset occurs if $||r|| < \rho$, that is, when the input-LTM matching is below the vigilance. If $||r|| < \rho$, learning takes place when the input-LTM match is above vigilance. (The match may not be perfect, but is close enough.) Then, update the LTM (bottom-up and top-down) traces.

Choose initial LTM traces for proper operation as follows.

By figure 4.13, if $||Z_J|| \to 0$, no reset occurs during learning. Thus, setting top-down LTM traces to

$$Z_{ji}(0) = 0 \tag{4.80}$$

enables initial learning.

Choose the initial bottom-up LTM traces to stabilize the category selection. The steady-state bottom-up LTM traces are

$$||Z^J|| \overset{t \to \infty}{\to} \frac{1}{1-d}. \tag{4.81}$$

To have $||Z^J||$ for a committed node larger than $||Z^J||$ for an uncommitted node, assume

$$||Z^J(0)|| \le \frac{1}{1-d}. \tag{4.82}$$

If $Z^J(0)$ is uniform,

$$0 < Z_{ij}(0) \leq \frac{1}{(1-d)\sqrt{M}}. \tag{4.83}$$

Thus, choose initial bottom-up LTM traces to satisfy the inequality. A common set of initial values is

$$Z_{ij}(0) = \frac{1}{(1-d)\sqrt{M}}. \tag{4.84}$$

In summary, the ART-2 NN is fairly complex. Nevertheless, simple examples can show its global behavior. The exercises give examples computable by hand.

The ART-2 algorithm has some arbitrariness. When to make the norm-to-threshold comparison is unclear for deciding reset. In practice the matching test is made before the F_1 STM reaches steady-state.

The adaptive-resonance-theoretic NNs are important for modeling and for applications. And many researchers expect their importance to increase relative to other kinds of NNs. Recently, ART-2A and ART-3 were introduced [16,17].

ART-2A is a version of ART-2 for large-scale neural computations. The operating principles of ART-2A are the same as ART-2.

ART-3 is a multilayer NN, that is, with F_1, F_2, ..., that models the biological synapse. Discussion of ART-3 is postponed until researchers develop its utility.

4.3 HOPFIELD NEURAL NETWORKS

The preceding ART NNs model biology. This section and the next develop two nonbiological NNs, Hopfield NNs and perceptrons. They are interesting because of their applications. These nonbiological NNs are special cases of the general theory developed in chapter 2.

Historically, the Hopfield NN regenerated interest in the field. This NN is popular with theoreticians because its simplicity allows for extended mathematical analyses. The Hopfield NN often serves to exhibit properties of NNs to new readers. Its applications, however, are limited because more powerful NNs are known.

Matrix notation is convenient for deriving the Hopfield NN. Let

$$x = (x_1, \ldots, x_N)^T \tag{4.85}$$

be a $N \times 1$ matrix associated with an N-element memory, where x is the STM trace, $x_i \in \Re$, and $(\ )^T$ is the transpose operation.

Let

$$z^i = (z_1^i, \ldots, z_N^i)^T \tag{4.86}$$

be the ith stored memory with N elements, where $z_j^i \in \Re$. z^i is a LTM trace. Assume M stored memories, given by the set $\{z^i\}_1^M$.

Construct a dynamic system with specified asymptotic properties as follows.

Starting from an initial vector, $x(0)$, the system is to relax to the nearest z^i. A metric measures closeness. Write the system symbolically as

$$\frac{dx}{dt} = f(x, z^1, \ldots, z^M), \tag{4.87}$$

where x is the dependent variable and $z^1, \ldots, z^M$ are parameters.

To show asymptotic properties, define a potential function, $P(x, z^1, \ldots, z^M)$, for the right-side of (4.87). Let

$$\frac{dP}{dx} = -f(x, z^1, \ldots, z^M), \tag{4.88}$$

where $P(\ )$ is a scalar. Matrix differentiation rules define dP/dx [20, p. 135].

To be stable $P(x)$ generally opens upward. The vectors $\{z^1, \ldots, z^M\}$ establish the minima of $P(x)$. The vectors are the asymptotic stable points of the system.

For example, a simple stable potential is the form

$$P(x, z^1, \ldots, z^M) = (a/2)x^T x + P'(x, z^1, \ldots, z^M), \tag{4.89}$$

where $P'(\ )$ is a perturbation from a reference quadratic potential.

The dynamic system is

$$\frac{dx}{dt} = -ax - \frac{dP'}{dx}. \tag{4.90}$$

The simplest system has a single memory ($M = 1$). Let

$$P(x, z^1, \ldots, z^M) = (a/2)x^T x + z^T x, \text{ for } a > 0, \tag{4.91}$$

giving

$$\frac{dx}{dt} = -ax + z. \tag{4.92}$$

This system relaxes to $x = z/a$ for every initial condition, $x(0)$, as shown in figure 4.14.

Construct a two memory system ($M = 2$) as follows.

$$\frac{dx}{dt} = -ax + C_1(x, z^1)z^1 + C_2(x, z^2)z^2, \tag{4.93}$$

where $C_1(\ ,\ )$ and $C_2(\ ,\ )$ are coefficients.

Choose $C_1(\ ,\ )$ to measure closeness of $x(t)$ to z^1. Assume $a = 1$ (equivalent to rescaling the variables). If $C_1 \gg C_2$, the system relaxes to z^1, as shown in figure 4.15.

A simple closeness measure is using the inner product of $sgn\ x$ and z^1. Applying an inner product, let

$$C_1(x, z^1) = (sgn\ x, z^1) = \sum_{i=1}^{N} (sgn\ x_i)z_i^1. \tag{4.94}$$

When $x = z^1$, (4.94) becomes

$$C_1(z^1, z^1) = (sgn\ z^1, z^1) = ||z_1^1||_1. \tag{4.95}$$

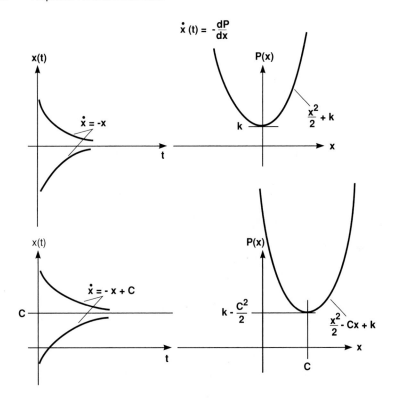

Figure 4.14   Two simple differential equations that are asymptotically stable and their potential functions. Stable potential functions are concave upward. Extension to finite dimensional systems is direct using matrix notation.

Many inner products are possible for $||z_1^1||$. The standard inner product gives

$$||z_1^1||_1 = \sum_{i=1}^{N} |z_i^1|, \tag{4.96}$$

which is the sum norm, or more picturesquely, the <u>Manhattan norm</u>.

When $x = z^2$, (4.94) becomes

$$C_1(z^2, z^1) = 0 \tag{4.97}$$

for uncorrelated coefficients of the memory vectors.

Defining $C_2(\ ,\ )$ in a similar way, these coefficients measure the closeness of $x(t)$ to each stored memory.

Generalizing to M memories, the system becomes

$$\frac{dx}{dt} = -ax + z^1(sgn\ x, z^1) + \ldots + z^M(sgn\ x, z^M). \tag{4.98}$$

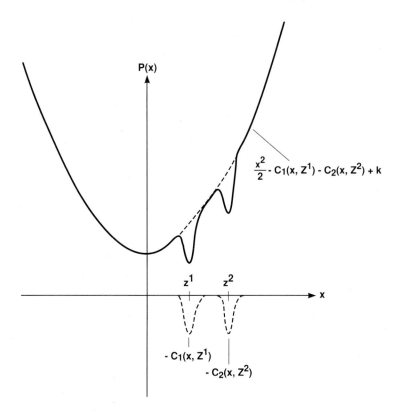

Figure 4.15   The Hopfield neural network constructs a potential that generally opens upward. To illustrate, consider two functions, (z_1, x) and (z_2, x). When x is close to z_1, (z_1, x) dominates over (z_2, x). Then, the system relaxes to z_1. Similar comments hold for z_2. As shown, the potential has local minima near the stored memories, z_1 and z_2. The potential, however, may have other (spurious) minima causing the system to relax to nonsense values.

Rewrite (4.98) exploiting the identities

$$z(sgn\ x, z) = (sgn\ x, z)z = (z^T sgn\ x)z = (zz^T)sgn\ x.$$

Factoring out $sgn\ x$ gives

$$\frac{dx}{dt} = -ax + (z^1 z^{1T} + \ldots + z^M z^{MT})sgn\ x. \tag{4.99}$$

The standard form of the Hopfield NN is

$$\frac{dx}{dt} = -ax + T sgn\ x, \tag{4.100}$$

where

$$T = \sum_{i=1}^{M} z^i z^{iT} \tag{4.101}$$

is the sum of the outer products of the stored memory vectors.

The perturbation potential is

$$\frac{dP'}{dx} = -T\,sgn\,x, \tag{4.102}$$

where $P'(x)$ opens downward. Adding $P'(x)$ to the upward-opening quadratic term produces local minima.

Some minima correspond to memories. Other minima are spurious stable points, that is, not vectors used in defining T.

Choose the coefficient a to normalize the memory lengths. As $x(t)$ approaches z^1, the system becomes

$$\frac{dx}{dt} = -ax + z^1 ||z^1||_1.$$

If $x(t) \to z^1$, $\frac{dx}{dt} \to 0$ for t large, giving

$$0 = -ax + z^1 ||z^1||_1.$$

Thus, $a = ||z^1||_1$. Similar comments hold for $z^2, \ldots, z^M$. Assuming all stored memories have the same length, setting $a = ||z^i||$ ensures convergence to the stored memory and not to a scalar multiple.

If $||z^i||$ is the same for all memory vectors, the memory vectors are distributed on the surface of an N-dimensional sphere. This is the simplex signal set in digital communication theory.

Other norms may be used. For example, the weighted norm

$$C_1(x, z) = (sgn\,x, z)_W = z^T W\,sgn\,x,$$

where W is positive definite, that is, a square matrix with positive real eigenvalues. This norm allows weighting the significance of each element. For example, the most significant bit (MSB) could be weighted more than the least significant bit (LSB).

Summarizing the properties of the Hopfield NN, the system from (4.98) is

$$\epsilon \dot{x}_i = -x + z^1(sgn\,x, z^1) + \ldots + z^M(sgn\,x_i, z^M). \tag{4.103}$$

If x is nearest to z^1 as measured by the sum norm,

$$\epsilon \dot{x}_i = -x + z^1(sgn\,z^1, z^1) + \ldots + z^M(sgn\,z^1, z^M)$$

and

$$\epsilon \dot{x} \approx -x + z^1(sgn\,z^1, z^1).$$

Or, $x(0) \to z^1$ as $t \to \infty$.

Computer simulation shows that to avoid convergence to a spurious minima,

$$M \le 0.15N. \tag{4.104}$$

That is, the stored memories are equal to or less than 15 percent of the elements.

Connecting the Hopfield NN with the general theory of chapter 2 is by manipulation. Write (4.103) in component form

$$\epsilon \dot{x}_i = -x_i + \sum_{j=1}^{N} t_{ij} sgn\, x_j. \tag{4.105}$$

Replace the $sgn(\ )$ function with a sigmoid function, that is,

$$sgn\, x_j \rightarrow f(x_j), \tag{4.106}$$

giving

$$\epsilon \dot{x}_i = -x_i + \sum_{j=1}^{N} t_{ij} f(x_j). \tag{4.107}$$

Let $f(x_j) = S_{ji}$ and $t_{ij} = Z_{ji}$. Then,

$$\epsilon \dot{x}_i = -x_i + \sum_{j=1}^{N} S_{ji} Z_{ji}, \tag{4.108}$$

which is the additive STM equation without external inputs derived in chapter 2.

Thus, derive the Hopfield NN by starting with the general additive STM equations, neglecting terms and making simplifications. Not vice versa.

Applications of the Hopfield NN follow from its properties and interpreting the inputs-outputs strings. First, if the initial vector, $x(0)$, is a message N-bits long with errors, the NN relaxes to the nearest correct message. That is, the Hopfield NN gives forward error correction (FEC) by operating as a decoder of a block-encoded message.

Second, if the initial vector is part of a stored memory, the NN relaxes to the nearest complete memory. That is, the NN is a content-addressable memory (CAM).

Third, if the initial vector is a memory trace, the NN relaxes to a different memory having to do with the input. That is, the NN is an associative memory.

4.4 PERCEPTRONS

Nonbiological NNs have many applications. The preceding Hopfield NN is one class of nonbiological NNs. Another class is perceptrons. The advantages of these nonbiological NNs lie in their use as calculation tools and not in the insight they give to neural operation.

Understanding perceptrons, however, is important for at least two reasons. First, perceptrons compose the majority of NNs today. For this reason they are a common reference for comparing NNs. Second, a researcher faced with meetings, discussions, and journal articles needs an understanding of perceptron basics and rules of thumb.

This section introduces perceptrons as follows. First, it develops the feedforward structure by a geometric approach for convex and nonconvex decision regions, multiple classification categories, and multidimensional inputs. Next, it shows that the most general perceptron has two hidden layers, and it discusses the classical exclusive OR (XOR) problem. Then, it discusses self-learning strategies to speed up the widely used backpropagation algorithm.

Consider specifying regions in a two-dimensional (2-D) space. Figure 4.16 shows a 2-D input space with Cartesian coordinates x_1 and x_2. A line separates two semi-infinite regions. To establish notation, assume the equation of the line is

$$w_1x_1 + w_2x_2 - \theta = 0. \tag{4.109}$$

The region to the right or below the line is

$$w_1x_1 + w_2x_2 - \theta > 0. \tag{4.110}$$

The region to the left or above the line is

$$w_1x_1 + w_2x_2 - \theta < 0.$$

Equivalently, this region is also

$$-w_1x_1 - w_2x_2 + \theta > 0. \tag{4.111}$$

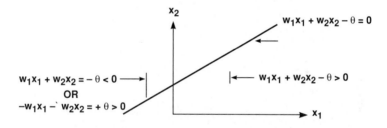

Figure 4.16   Semi-infinite regions in two dimensions. Replacing the equal sign by an inequality in the equation for a line defines regions to the left or right.

In the following treatment, the $>$ inequality is convenient, so equations (4.110) and (4.111) are used. Note that except for the sign, (4.110) and (4.111) are the same.

For example, figure 4.17 shows a triangular region R. Region R, a set of points (x_1, x_2), satisfies three inequalities of the forms of (4.110). That is, region R is right of line 1 and above line 2 and left of line 3. In defining line 1, line 2, and line 3, choose the signs of the coefficients so that the terms are positive in the inequalities.

Thus, write R as

$$R = \{(x_1, x_2) | (w_{11}x_1 + w_{12}x_2 + \theta_1 > 0)$$
$$\bigcap (w_{21}x_1 + w_{22}x_2 + \theta_2 > 0) \tag{4.112}$$
$$\bigcap (w_{31}x_1 + w_{32}x_2 + \theta_3 > 0)\},$$

where $\bigcap$ is the logical AND (intersection) operator.

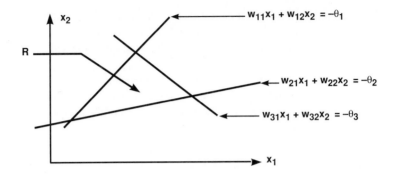

Figure 4.17 Specifying a finite region in two dimensions. To apply to neural networks, use set notation and greater-than inequalities.

Figure 4.18 shows a network implementing (4.112). Each summation node generates a line. The unit step function, $\Pi(\ )$, gives the inequality, where $\Pi(0) = 1$. A three-input AND gate gives the intersection operation. Note, the biases, θ, map a zero input to a nonzero output.

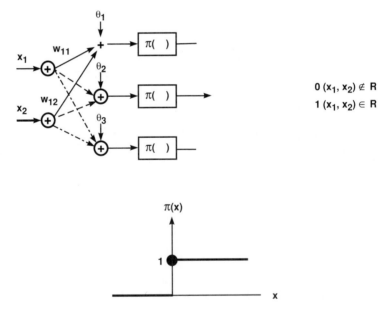

Figure 4.18 A network for a triangular region in two dimensions. Three in-equalities, represented by the three paths in the network, define the region. The parameters, w_{11}, w_{12}, θ_1, define one of three lines bounding the region. A unit step function, $\pi(\ )$ defines the inequality. If the input point (x_1, x_2) lies in the region, the logic AND gate produces an output 1. Otherwise, the output is 0.

Figure 4.19 shows a NN implementing a three-input AND gate. The biases are in the interval $[-3, -2)$.

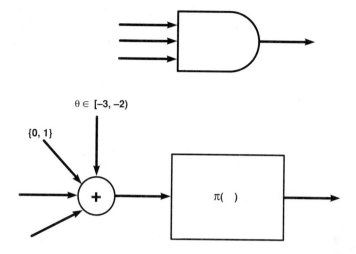

$\theta \in [-3, -2)$

$\{0, 1\}$

$\pi(\ )$

Figure 4.19   Perceptron implementation of a three-input logic AND gate. Inputs are 0 or 1. Because of a bias θ in the range $-3 \geq \theta < 2$ and a unit step function, the output is 1 if and only if all three inputs are 1. Otherwise, the output is 0.

Combining figures 4.18 and 4.19 gives a NN for 2-D triangular decision regions, shown in figure 4.20. Three layers can be identified: (1) an INPUT layer, (2) a PLANE layer, and (3) an AND layer. The AND layer is the OUTPUT layer for this NN. Figure 4.20 shows the neurons for each layer. By adding neurons to the PLANE layer, this NN is sufficient for every finite simply connected region.

A first extension is to arbitrarily shaped regions. First, assume two separate regions, shown in figure 4.21. Region R_1 is a triangular region. Region R_2 is a semi-infinite region to the left of two lines. Assume points in both regions belong to a region called R.

Then, inequalities define R as

$$R = \{(x_1, x_2) \mid \bigcap_{j=1}^{3} (w_{j1}x_1 + w_{j2}x_2 + \theta_j > 0)$$
$$\bigcup (\bigcap_{j=4}^{5} (w_{j1}x_1 + w_{j2}x_2 + \theta_j > 0)\}, \tag{4.113}$$

where $\bigcup$ is the logical OR (union) operation.

Figure 4.21 shows a NN implementing (4.113). The OR gate is simply a summation with a smaller bias than for an AND gate.

In figure 4.22, four layers define an arbitrary decision region. The OR layer acts as the OUTPUT layer. Moreover, no classification task takes more than four layers (two hidden layers), because every expression in mathematical logic is expressible in conjunction normal form.

While four layers are enough for an arbitrary nonconvex region, in general the minimum layers may be less than four. The AND-OR layers can often be combined in a single layer consisting of a bias and a summation.

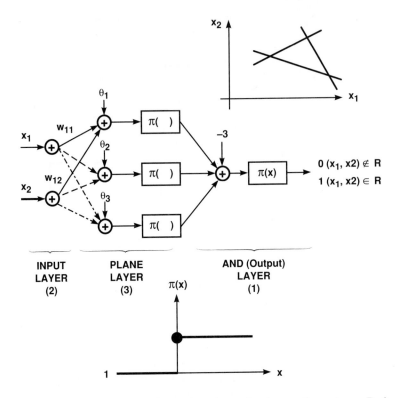

Figure 4.20 A perceptron for a triangular region in two dimensions. Each summing node-step function represents an idealized neuron (node), which first multiples inputs by the weights and then if above a threshold, produces an output 1. As shown, this example has six nodes and three layers. The first layer is the input layer. The second layer, called the plane layer, defines lines (planes) bounding the region. The third layer, called the AND layer, has the logic AND and is also the output layer.

Figure 4.23 shows a nonconvex region realized by three layers using appropriate biases and weights [50]. For 2-D this simplification can be frequently found. Simplification with higher dimensional inputs is more difficult. And while three-layer NNs are possible, equivalent four-layer NNs are easily constructed and interpreted.

A second extension is discriminating many classes.

Figure 4.24 shows the decision regions for three classes. Define each class by the INPUT-PLANE-AND-OUTPUT(OR) architecture. By this approach, three classes (and their negation) lead to three neurons in the OUTPUT layer.

A third extension is to higher dimensional inputs. Figure 4.25 shows a slab in 3-D space, specified by two inequalities. A 3-D cube is the intersection (AND) of three slabs. Thus, a cubic decision region in 3-D input space leads to the network shown in figure 4.26. To define the decision region, fix the weights and adjust the biases. Extension to higher

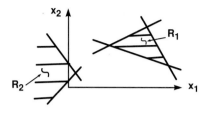

$$R = \{(x_1, x_2) | \overset{3}{\underset{j=1}{\cap}} (w_{j1}x_1 + w_{j2}x_2 + \theta_j > 0)$$

$$\cup [\overset{5}{\underset{j=4}{\cap}} (w_{j1}x_1 + w_{j2}x_2 + \theta_j > 0)]\}$$

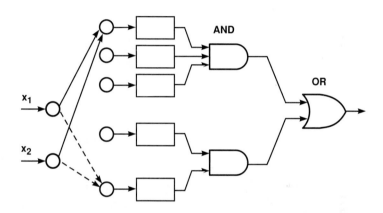

Figure 4.21   A network for two regions, R_1 and R_2. R_1 is a triangular region defined as in figure 4.20. R_2 is a semi-infinite region defined by two lines, or two paths in the network. If the input point (x_1, x_2) lies in either region, the logic OR gate produces 1. Otherwise, the output is 0.

dimensional decision regions is direct and involves the intersection of planes defined in the input space.

The XOR problem is historically significant in perceptron theory. Minsky and Papert [71] critiqued the two-layer perceptron on its failure to solve the XOR problem. To the author's knowledge, however, this multilayer perceptron theory was not known when the objection was made.

Figure 4.27 shows the XOR problem in the present notation. The XOR operator classifies points (1,0) and (0,1) as "one" and other points as "zero." A NN defines regions containing (1,0) and (0,1). Figure 4.28 shows square regions around the points. The decision region, R, consists of R_1 and R_2. That is,

$$R = \{(x_1, x_2) | (x_1, x_2) \in R_1 \bigcup (x_1, x_2) \in R_2\}. \tag{4.114}$$

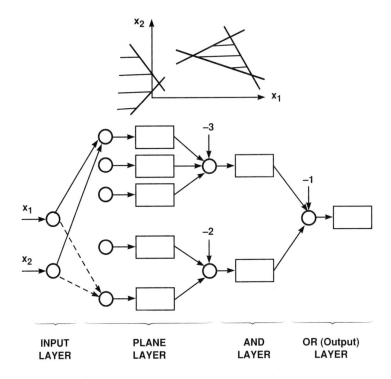

Figure 4.22   A perceptron for the region shown in figure 4.21. For clarity some
connections are not shown. A node with threshold -2 implements the two-input
logic OR gate. In general, four layers is the maximum number of layers needed
for an input space, although fewer layers are sometimes adequate (see figure
4.23).

In the notation of figure 4.28, (4.114) becomes

$$R = \{(x_1, x_2) | (x_1 > 1 - \epsilon \bigcap x_1 > 1 + \epsilon \bigcap x_2 > -\epsilon \bigcap x_2 < \epsilon)$$

$$\bigcup (x_1 > -\epsilon \bigcap x_1 < \epsilon \bigcap x_2 > 1 - \epsilon \bigcap x_2 > 1 + \epsilon)\}. \qquad (4.115)$$

Figure 4.29 shows a NN implementation of (4.114). As seen, the NN needs 13 neurons
in four layers.

Figure 4.30 shows a simpler XOR solution. The decision region is defined by two
lines. The NN has five neurons in three layers.

Thus, a solution to XOR depends on how the output is defined for inputs not 0 or 1.
So the XOR solution is not unique, and many solutions are possible.

The geometric description of perceptrons suggests many learning algorithms. Two
simple self-learning algorithms follow. Assume a 2-D input space. A simple algorithm
uses a set of training points to define a rectangular decision region for class 1. Figure 4.31
shows implementing this region with four neurons with fixed known weights. The biases
are adjusted to enclose the region.

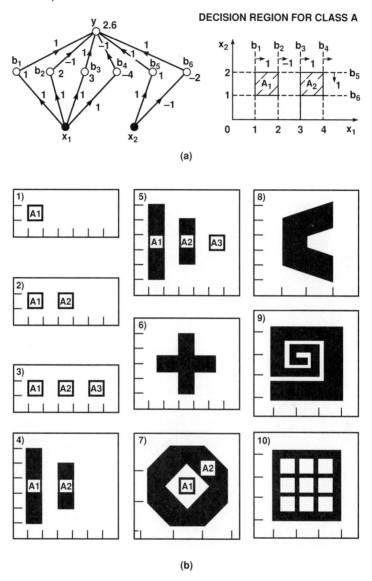

Figure 4.23 (a) A three-layer perceptron forming disjoint regions for class A (shaded areas). The left part shows connection weights and node biases. Dashed lines show the lines formed by nodes. Arrows point to the half plane where the node outputs are 1. (b) Ten example regions formed by three-layer perceptrons.

Let the set $\{x_1(k), x_2(k)\}$ with $k = 1, \ldots, N$ be N training points. The biases $\theta_1, \theta_1', \ldots, \theta_4, \theta_4'$ are from

$$\theta_1 = \max_k \{x_1(k)\} \qquad (4.116)$$

and

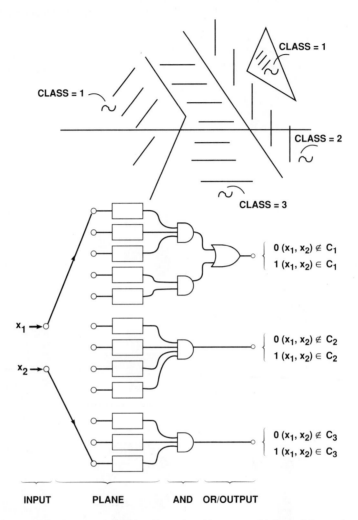

Figure 4.24 A network for two-dimensional inputs, multiple decision regions, and three classes, illustrating extension of network in figure 4.21.

$$\theta_1' = \min_k \{x_1(k)\}. \tag{4.117}$$

To implement (4.116) in a recursive way, assume $\theta_1(k+1)$ is from the inequalities

$$x_1(k) - \theta_1(k) \begin{cases} > 0, & \theta_1(k+1) = x_1(k) \\ \leq 0, & \theta_1(k+1) = \theta_1(k). \end{cases} \tag{4.118}$$

Equivalently, $\theta_1(k)$ is by

$$\theta_1(k+1) = y\theta_1(k) + (1-y)x_1(k), \tag{4.119}$$

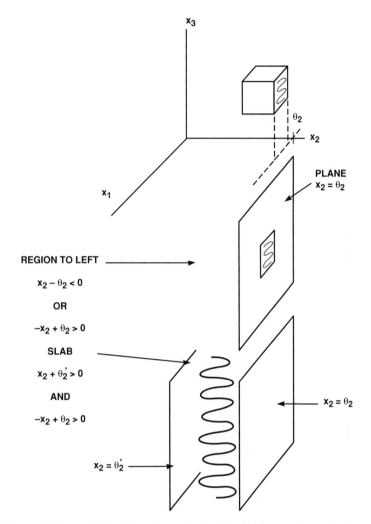

Figure 4.25 Specifying three-dimensional slabs. Replacing the equal sign by an inequality in the equation for a plane that is perpendicular to a coordinate axis defines a volume to the left or right. Combining two inequalities defines a slab.

where

$$y = \Pi(-x_1 + \theta_1). \tag{4.120}$$

Figure 4.32 shows computing y by the system, then computing $\theta_1(k + 1)$ by a first-order feedback system. This approach leads to a learning feedback system, shown in figure 4.33.

Another self-learning strategy is to bound a simply connected decision region by straight lines produced in a stepwise fashion. Figure 4.34 shows the idea. Start with three points to form a triangle. Add a fourth training point. If the fourth point is in the triangle,

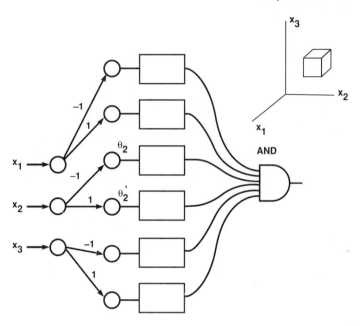

Figure 4.26   A network for a parallelopiped region in three dimensions. As shown, the thresholds define the sides. The logic AND gate has six inputs. All inputs must be 1 if the input point (x_1, x_2, x_3) lies in the region.

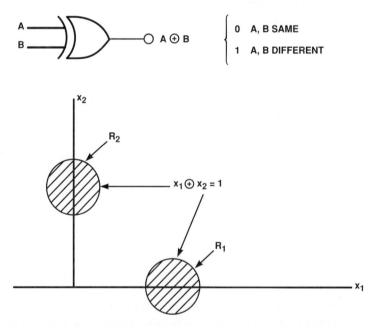

Figure 4.27   XOR definition. The logic XOR gate produces 0 if all inputs are the same. Otherwise, it produces 1. For two dimensions, define regions R_1 and R_2 as shown. For an XOR network, inputs lying in R_1 and R_2 produce 1.

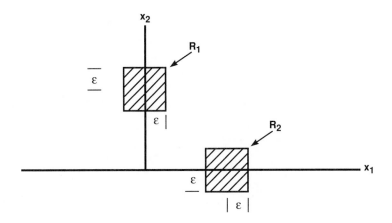

Figure 4.28   Decision region for the XOR problem illustrating regions R_1 and R_2 defined by lines perpendicular to the coordinate axes.

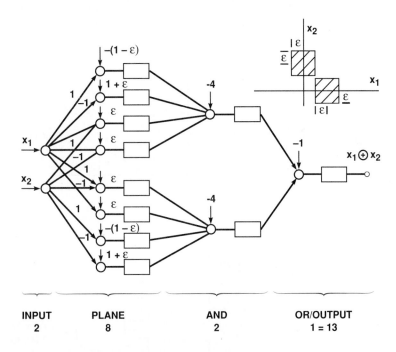

Figure 4.29   A perceptron for the XOR problem with regions from figure 4.28. The network has 13 nodes arranged in four layers.

no change is made. If the point is outside the triangle, change the region to four-sided by adding another neuron.

The decision region changes to that shown in figure 4.35. As more points are added, there is a neuron in the second layer for every line. The lower figure shows alternate decision regions for the same training set. That is, the solution is not unique.

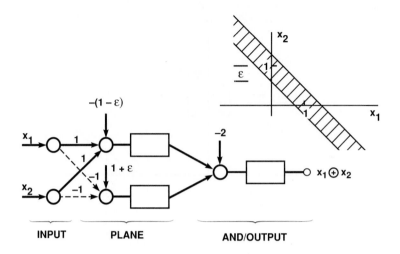

Figure 4.30   A perceptron for the XOR problem with regions defined by two lines. The network has five nodes arranged in three layers.

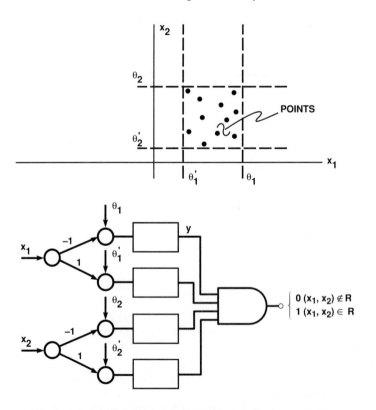

Figure 4.31   A simple two-dimensional region enclosing a set of points and the corresponding network. The biases define the lines.

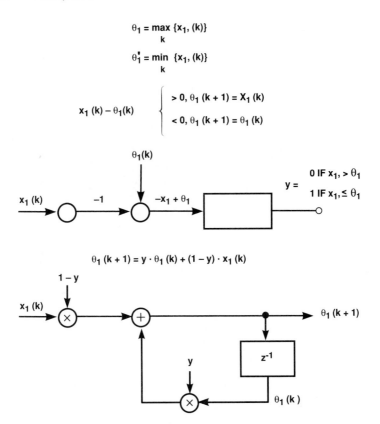

$$\theta_1 = \max_k \{x_1, (k)\}$$

$$\theta_1^{\cdot} = \min_k \{x_1, (k)\}$$

$$x_1(k) - \theta_1(k) \quad \begin{cases} > 0, \theta_1(k+1) = X_1(k) \\ \\ < 0, \theta_1(k+1) = \theta_1(k) \end{cases}$$

$$\theta_1(k+1) = y \cdot \theta_1(k) + (1-y) \cdot x_1(k)$$

Figure 4.32   Update system illustrating simple feedback to adjust biases. An input x_1 at time index k, $x_1(k)$ produces output y, shown in figure 4.31. The input $x_1(k)$ is also sent to another system to produce the updated bias $\theta_1(k+1)$.

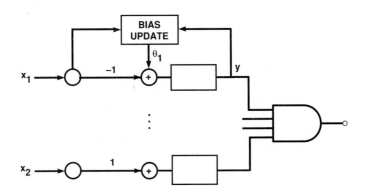

Figure 4.33   Combining networks of figures 4.31 and 4.32 gives a network that automatically adjusts biases. During a training period, an input dataset passes through the system to set the biases. After training, the perceptron classifies other inputs.

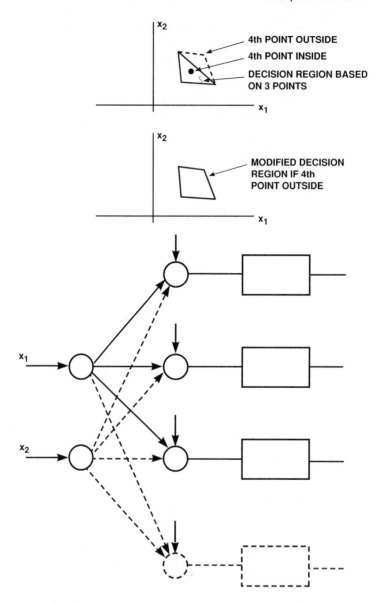

Figure 4.34 A perceptron that adjusts the nodes in the plane layer. During training on an input dataset, if a, say, fourth point lies outside of the region for a class, the output is 0. Adding another node to the plane layer changes the region, as shown.

Figure 4.36 summarizes the general structure of perceptrons. That is, the architecture consists of four layers: INPUT-PLANE-AND-OUTPUT(OR). Two layers are hidden. Three layers have coefficients defining one or more decision regions. Figure 4.36 shows the neurons in each layer.

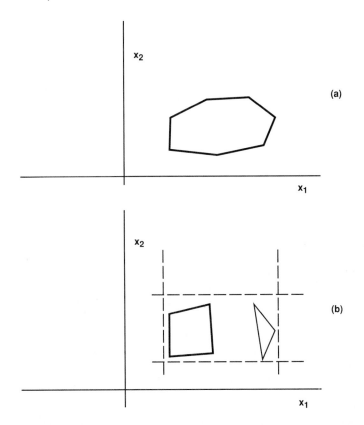

Figure 4.35   Evolution of the region with more training inputs. (a) Adding nodes to the plane layer produces a region bounded by lines. (b) Alternatively, with the same training dataset, adjusting the biases produces a region with sides perpendicular to the coordinate axes.

Currently, the most widely used method of setting the weights and biases is the generalized delta algorithm known as backpropagation [79, ch. 8]. In the backpropagation algorithm, the weights and biases in the three adjustable layers (PLANE-AND-OR) are set to small random values at first. A training set recursively adjusts the weights. Practice shows many iterations are needed. For example, a three-layer NN (one hidden layer) with 15-30-1 neurons typically needs over 100, 000 iterations before reaching steady state.

The geometric viewpoint, however, suggests prior knowledge about the classification problem can structure the NN, estimate coefficients, and develop new learning algorithms. (For a related approach, see [10] which describes using Voronoi diagrams—a partition of the space into convex regions.)

Finally, other extensions, not discussed, include use of sigmoid rather than step functions, and nonlinear functions of the input coordinates to form, say, spherical decision regions. Indeed, the geometric viewpoint gives a convenient baseline for understanding perceptron NNs and further work.

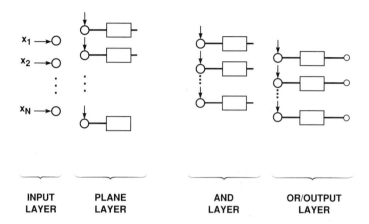

| INPUT | PLANE | AND | OR/OUTPUT |
| LAYER | LAYER | LAYER | LAYER |

Figure 4.36 General structure of perceptrons in four layers. While algorithms, such as backpropagation, can define biases and weights in each layer, insight into the application may produce a perceptron design faster and better.

SUGGESTED REFERENCES

B. KOSKO, *Unsupervised Learning in Noise*. This paper considers the stability of neural networks when structure is perturbed. Structural stability may be affected by thermal noise processes, electromagnetic interactions, and component failures. The stability properties can also be affected by unmodeled electrochemical and molecular processes in, say, synapses. The paper considers adaptive and nonadaptive neural networks, such as ART-2 and Hopfield NNs. One result is that if the processes ignored in the state equations produce a net random effect, their effect is unimportant to the global computations.

W. BROGAN, *Modern Control Theory*. Many elaborate treatises exist on temporal stability. Chapter 14 of this reference is a good summary. Section 14.6 contains material on the Lyapunov method.

G. CARPENTER AND S. GROSSBERG, *A Massively Parallel Architecture for a Self-Organizing Neural Pattern Recognition Machine*. References in previous chapters discuss the ART NNs. Indeed, the ART literature is rapidly increasing. Nearly every book on neural networks devotes some time to it. This paper is well known, and it is the fullest exposition of ART-1. It treats many advanced topics. A set of theorems summarize ART-1 properties. For example, a theorem shows that the order of input patterns is unimportant in training ART-1. Moreover, the coding is stable, with the LTM traces oscillating at most once because of learning. The paper gives an example of learning alphabet symbols.

R. LIPPMANN, *Introduction to Computing with Neural Networks*. This overview article discusses ART-1. It describes results from MIT Lincoln Laboratory studies. After training on "perfect inputs," if a noisy input is applied, the ART-1 will classify it with a similar example. Updating the LTM then degrades this LTM. More noisy inputs cause further growth of noisy LTMs. Possible improvements include adapting the LTM more slowly, or changing the vigilance.

S. GROSSBERG, *Studies of Mind and Brain*. ART was originated by Grossberg. Carpenter and Grossberg and others then developed ART NNs to the point where they are some of the most powerful known. Chapter 1 of this reference discusses the modeling with ART of environmentally driven and behaviorally meaningful code development.

G. CARPENTER AND S. GROSSBERG, *ART 2: Self-Organization of Stable Category Recognition Codes for Analog Input Patterns*. This is the best treatment of the ART-2 algorithm, and it is a classic paper in the field. It contains much information, especially the parameter sensitivity studies.

J. HOPFIELD, *Neural Networks and Physical Systems with Emergent Collective Computational Abilities*. This is a NN classic. The paper discusses associative memory by systems with many simple components (neurons). Hopfield and his associates developed this class of NNs and applied it to problems such as the traveling salesman problem. The major impact of the paper, however, was in producing interest in the field, which led to more powerful NNs.

K. PASSINO, *Neural Computing for Numeric-to-Symbolic Conversion in Control Systems*. Perceptrons have many applications. In this paper a perceptron is a numeric-to-symbolic convert for a discrete-event system controller. The controller supervises a continuous variable dynamic system. Several examples are given. The paper sets the biases and weights as described in the text. In this paper the technique is referred to as "Harvey's method." The method is an alternative way to speed up the well-known backpropagation algorithm.

EXERCISES

1. Assume the following:

   a. An ART-1 neural network with $M = 3$, $N = 5$, shown in figure 4.37.
   b. A set of consistent parameters and choose an initial set of LTMs.
   c. Training inputs $I(1) = (110)$, $I(2) = (011)$.
   d. Fast learning and other parameters.

   Compute the LTMs after a single training sequence cycle. What are the classifications of $I(3) = (100)$, $I(4) = (001)$, and $I(5) = (010)$?

2. What are the classifications of $I(3) = (100)$, $I(4) = (001)$, and $I(5) = (010)$ after this training sequence?

3. Let I_i be the ith input to ART-2. Assume zero top-down LTM trace. Find the noise threshold that attenuates I_i.

4. Let a saw-tooth input be presented to ART-2 varying between I_1 and I_2, with $I_1 < I_2$. Find the ratio I_2/I_1 so I_1 is stored as zero.

5. Show that multiples of the input to ART-2 are indistinguishable.

6. Show how the magnitude of the LTM trace varies with input pattern length.

7. Consider a medical diagnosis application of ART-2. Assume there are 25 characteristics, each with 5 values or levels, which are collected during interviews and observations of a patient. Assume some characteristics are critical for making a correct diagnosis, while some characteristics are not applicable for particular diagnoses. Design, describe the training, and outline the use of an ART-2 that recognizes patterns of input characteristics in 5 diagnostic categories (see [43] for a nursing diagnosis example). How could the system be updated with new information? How could the system be verified (algorithm correct), validated (agrees with reality), and accredited (accepted for use by practitioners)?

8. Design a Hopfield associative memory to store two memories, $I(1) = (110)$ and $I(2) = (011)$.

9. Show $I(1)$ and $I(2)$ are stable points.

10. Let $I(3) = (100)$. Show it relaxes to $I(1)$.

11. Design a multilayer perceptron to classify $I(1) = (110)$ and $I(2) = (011)$ in different categories.

12. Let $I(3) = (100)$. In what category is $I(3)$ classified?

5

Vision Systems

The first four chapters presented elementary NN modules. In the lateral interaction modules, we have controllers, feature detectors, and front-end processors. In the perceptron networks, we have simple classifiers. And in the ART networks, we have general memory units. This chapter applies these elementary modules to design machine vision systems that roughly model biology.

5.1 OVERVIEW OF HUMAN VISION

The plan of this chapter is to approach vision from a biological point of view. This section summarizes primate vision.

Vision here means higher primate vision, especially human vision. Although data are available for several species, many results come from the macaque monkey, an animal with visual capabilities like those of human beings. In comparison, the vision systems for creatures lower than primates differ significantly from primate vision.

The visual pathway from the eye goes to the visual cortex in two steps, shown in figure 5.1. The output from each retina divides at the optic chiasm and ends on neurons in the lateral geniculate nucleus (LGN). In turn the LGN axons project along the optic radiation to the visual cortex.

Table 1.5 summarizes characteristics of human vision. The retina has about 1.25×10^8 receptors. Processing in the retina compresses the data about 125 to 1. Thus, the resolution near fovea, the most sensitive part of the retina, is about 1000×1000 pixels.

The relative discrimination to brightness variations is 570 "just noticeable differences." Discrimination of frequency variations is 128 "just noticeable differences."

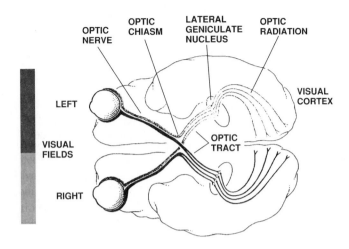

Figure 5.1   The underview of the human brain showing the visual pathways. For each retina, half of the axons go to the right tract, and the other half go to the left tract. (From Kuffler, et al. *From Neuron to Brain*. Reprinted by permission of Sinauer Associates, Inc., 1984).

The field of view (FOV) of each pixel is about 0.5 minutes of arc (8 millidegrees) at fovea with good contrast and brightness [51, p. 45]. Thus, the FOV of each eye for the highest acuity is 500 minutes of arc, or 8.3°. Moreover, the eyes can track with a precision of about 1 minute of arc [51, p. 34].

Assuming typical values of 7 bits per pixel and a 100 Hz pulse frequency along the optic nerve, the data rate to the visual cortex is about 700 Mb/s, less than the capacity of current fiber optic channels.

Pathway characteristics of key brain areas in vision, shown in figure 5.2, are as follows. Research shows vision involves at least a dozen cortical areas in primates [83, p. 371]. Moreover, the vision system has a hierarchical structure. That is, researchers can assign distinct processing levels to the modules making up the system. (Deductively, there is no reason to expect such organization. For example, the brain could be a complex network without distinct hierarchical levels [83, p. 371].)

Researchers have mapped over 30 pathways among vision-related areas. The number of actual pathways is probably much larger because many connections have not been studied. A basic finding is that most pathways connect the areas in reciprocal fashion [83, p. 371].

For the dozen visual areas, the overall cortical hierarchy has six levels. Researchers constructed the hierarchy by assigning each area to a level just above the highest area providing an input [83, p. 372]. The procedure leads to the six levels.

Architectural characteristics of vision processing are as follows. Anatomical, behavioral, and physiological data reveal two distinct channels for locating and classifying, shown in figure 5.2 by the dotted line and the X-Y pathways. The two channels separate at the retina and have separate retinal detector cells, labeled X and Y. They remain separate at the cortical and midbrain levels.

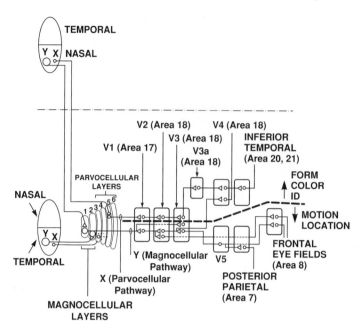

Figure 5.2   Schematic of visual projections to the brain areas involved in vision. (From Kandel and Schwartz. *Principles of Neural Science.* Adapted, with permission, from the *Annual Review of Neuroscience* Vol. 2, 1979, E. Kandel, and Appleton & Lange, 1985).

Evidence shows the classification channel analyzes form and color. The location channel analyzes visual motion across the FOV [85, p. 372].

The X-cells go to the classification channel [5, p. 353]. They are medium-sized cells with small optical fields which give high acuity and comparatively slow response times.

The Y-cells go to the location channel. They are big cells with large optical fields which give low acuity and fast response times.

(The W-cells, a third kind of retinal cell, go to the midbrain areas. The W-cells have small fields. They coordinate the FOV to head and eye movements. The population distribution is about 50 percent for X, 5 percent for Y, and 45 percent for W.)

The classification channel works as follows. The classification channel starts at the X-cells of the retina. The channel then goes to the retinal ganglion cell (RGC). It continues to the LGN, to the primary visual cortex (Vl—also called area 17), and the secondary visual cortex (V2–V5—also called area 18). It then goes to the inferior temporal cortex (ITC—also called areas 20 and 21).

The visual pathway maps the FOV seen by the eyes onto Vl. The mapping to Vl impresses the FOV on the fourth layer—of six layers—of the cortex sheet. The mapping is continuous, has the well-known logarithmic distortion near fovea, and rotates the external image about the horizontal axis, as shown next.

Figures 5.3 and 5.4 illustrate the mapping of the external FOV onto V1. In figure 5.3 (top), the external image has horizontal and vertical lines with a circle around the origin.

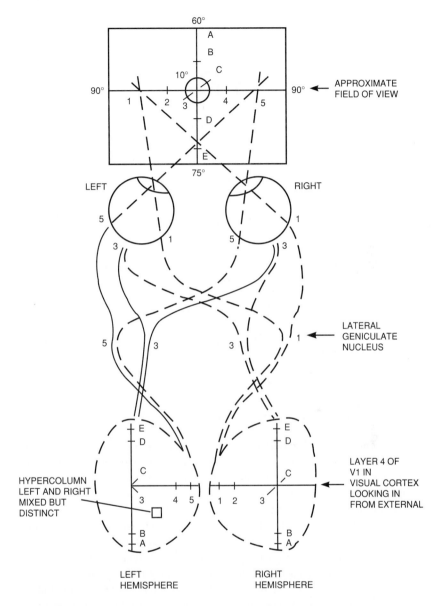

Figure 5.3   Retinotopic mapping of the visual field of view to the striate cortex. The mapping distorts and rotates the image about the horizontal axis. The right-eye view corresponds to the left cortex hemisphere, and vice versa. Distortion causes magnification near fovea. (Adapted from Frisby, 1980)

The figure numbers positions 1 through 5 along the horizontal line. The figure also marks positions A through E along the vertical. The circle has a radius of 8°, the FOV for highest acuity without moving the eyes.

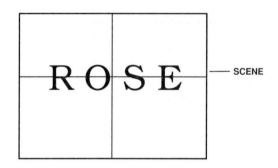

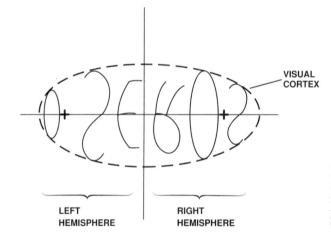

Figure 5.4   Example of the retinotopic mapping. The retinal image maintains its structure as the pathways transfer the pattern of stimulation from the retina to the striate cortex.

In figure 5.3 (bottom), crossover connections map the right-hand FOV of the two eyes to the left-side of V1 (as seen from the rear of the head). The mapping also interlaces the images from the two eyes. The images remain separate. Similarly, crossover connections map the left-hand FOV of the two eyes to the right-side of V1. The mapping also rotates the image about the horizontal axis.

Figure 5.3 shows magnification of the image. The mapping expands the region near the fovea, the region of highest acuity. For example, the distance from 3 to 4 and from 4 to 5 are equal in the external image. In V1 the distance from 3 to 4 is greater than from 4 to 5. Similarly, remarks hold for distances along the vertical.

Figure 5.4 shows the mapping of a word and the mapping of radial and circular lines. The mapping distorts and rotates the V1 image for a single eye. Circles in the external image get mapped to near vertical lines, and external radial lines get mapped to near horizontal lines. Measurements show the mapping is like a complex logarithm function.

The vision feature detectors work as follows. Areas V1, V2, and V3 function as feature detectors. As discovered by Hubel and Weisel (1955) [51], the features give contour and orientation information about the pattern.

Researchers have measured the response of individual cells (neurons) along the classification channel to external images [51, p. 69]. In the retina and LGN, the response is on-center/off-surround or off-center/on-surround. In Vl, three cell types have been found: simple, complex, and hypercomplex.

Simple cells respond to stationary edges, slits, or lines in the external image at precise orientation angles. In human beings the angular resolution between two straight lines is about $10°$ [30, p. 48]. Interpolation allows discrimination between two lines differing by about $3°$. A stationary line must be carefully oriented and positioned to produce a response from a simple cell.

The <u>receptive field</u> of a V1 neuron is a small area of the retina on which light must fall to affect the neuron. At fovea simple cells have receptive fields measuring about $\frac{1}{4}°$ by $\frac{1}{4}°$. At the periphery, the receptive field size is about $1°$ by $1°$.

Complex cells respond to moving edges, slits, or lines in a precise direction. About 75 percent of cells in Vl are complex [51, p. 74]. The receptive field of complex cells is slightly larger than that for simple cells. Near fovea the receptive field size is about $\frac{1}{2}°$ by $\frac{1}{2}°$.

Hypercomplex cells respond if one or two ends of a line stop in the receptive area. If the line goes through the receptive area without stopping, the hypercomplex cell response goes to 0 or to a constant value.

Summarizing the feature detectors, the features in primate vision are stationary or moving edges, slots, or lines. In comparison, these are not the features commonly used in current machine vision (MV) algorithms. Typical features in MV algorithms are corners, faces, frequencies, or responses of matched filters.

(Although a global Fourier transformed by the visual cortex was hypothesized erroneously, research shows a local spatial frequency analysis starting in the striate cortex [60,74]. This analysis is done by interactions among adjacent simple cells.)

The ITC (areas 20 and 21) in the classification channel works like a classifier. The ITC output goes to higher level centers of logic and emotion [53, ch. 5]. The location channel works as follows.

A location channel starts at the Y-cells of the retina. The channel goes through the midbrain areas to the superior colliculus (SC) and then to the pulvinar nucleus (PT). It then goes to the posterior parietal (PP). The output of this channel goes to the frontal eye fields (area 8). Evidence suggests this system is responsible for location analyses of objects in the FOV.

Interconnections link the classification and location channels. The SC projects directly to the ITC, bypassing the rest of the main route. The PT projects to the secondary visual cortices and to the ITC. The classification channel also passes data to the location channel by paths from Vl to the SC and to the PT [53, p. 101].

Considering the system as a whole, researchers believe it works as follows. Retinal images send data for pattern analysis by the classification channel. The classifying system passes the data from RGC to LGN to Vl, then through paths in V2, V3, V4, and V5, and then to the ITC.

At the same time, retinal images pass through midbrain routes that locate objects and analyze spatial relations and motion. Moreover, the location system interacts with the pattern analysis system at most steps along the route. Key interactions occur in the location visual cortex for constructing spatial relations [53, p. 101].

Besides the level scheme, a relationship exists between the level and the receptive field size.

Receptive fields are smallest in Vl. The fields increase in size at successive levels of the hierarchy [83, p. 372]. Researchers also found that receptive field parameters—size, shape, and location—vary [53, ch. 5]. That is, a mechanism, probably presynaptic inhibition, adaptively adjusts a feature detecting cell. (Presynaptic inhibition is a mechanism that acts to turn off selected inputs to a neuron—see chapter 2.)

Presynaptic inhibition in the feature detection stages changes the shape and location of the receptive field. Under normal conditions, stimulating the ITC changes the receptive fields of area Vl, suggesting that the ITC may exert feedback control over the feature detectors. Moreover, emotional states also alter the receptive fields.

Thus, recognition is likely an active feedback process that restructures the feature extraction stages. That is, feedforward and feedback signals continue until matching an input and some known class of stimulus [53, p. 108].

Recognition starts with standard receptive fields. If matching by the ITC fails, feedback shifts the processes in the preceding stages to extract features for another object class.

Research also suggests a mechanism for directing attention to selected locations in the FOV. In short, windowing occurs.

Windowing focuses on small details and ends notice of other objects in the FOV. Researchers suspect that the midbrain directs this process, perhaps cued by cortical inputs.

The vision system has other inputs besides those from the retina. Signals from the motor systems give data about eye position. Moreover, inputs from the frontal cortex may be the source of selective attention. These attention inputs direct goal-related processes.

Visual memory is another source of input, which may improve the search strategy in the perceptual analysis [53, p. 132].

Research shows considerable use of feedforward signals. Outputs of the visual front end supply a variety of later stages. Indeed, the higher processing levels may tap the early stages for simple data, such as overall brightness.

Output from each stage of processing is probably available to all parts of the system. The primary cortex, however, gives information about the detailed nature of the visual field and its spatial structure. The primary cortex does not analyze patterns into objects. To organize patterns, the higher levels draw on experience, that is memory.

After visual processing, the brain uses outputs from the visual system throughout. One area records visual objects (memory). Another area organizes a logical world model from experience and sensory inputs (cognition). Yet another area responds emotionally to perceived objects (motivation) [53, ch. 5].

The system is asynchronous, that is, it has no master clock. The system is a serial-parallel, analog, asynchronous, real-time computing machine. In comparison man-made computers are mostly serial, digital, synchronous, and off-line.

The system continually updates on each pathway. Thus, there will be differences among the modules in the processing time, in the spatial relations of FOV objects, and in the external representation of the external world. In short, spatial-temporal smearing occurs (see chapter 9 for further discussion).

In practice the longest times are a fraction of a second, roughly, the characteristic visual interaction time with the outside world.

Summarizing the above description, figure 5.5 shows a block diagram of the brain's visual processing. The system is a sensor-preprocessor-feature-extracting-classifier system. A small number of serial stages move large arrays of data. In each stage the processing is heavily parallel. Feedforward and feedback pathways connect the modules.

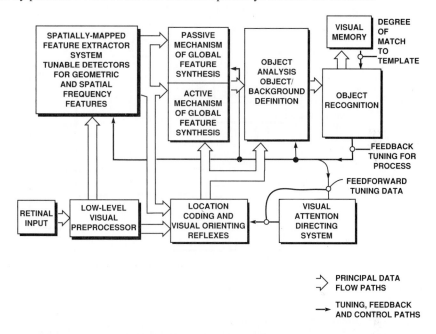

Figure 5.5   A block diagram of the vision system containing modules. (From Kent. *The Brains of Men and Machines*. Reprinted with permission of E. Kent, 1981).

5.2 AN ARCHITECTURE FOR MACHINE VISION

Research suggests that the advantages of biological vision over current MV are from feedback, flexible control, and the kinds of feature detectors. This section describes an example general purpose MV system having some of these biological characteristics.

The purpose of the system is to find and identify spatial patterns of luminance in the FOV. The term "general purpose" means recognizing objects of different classes without changing the algorithm. Applying the system means setting a few sensitivity parameters and training by examples.

The design method is to model the human vision system. The functions of the modules approximate those of the human brain. For convenience, implementation in a testbed (described below) uses a mixture of NNs and standard processing algorithms.

The system recognizes gray images in the FOV, with arbitrary translations and rotations. It does not emulate certain biological characteristics. Not emulated are binocularity, size invariance, motion perception, color sensitivity, and discernment of virtual boundaries. Indeed, many applications can omit these properties.

The architecture of the system has location and classification channels that work together. The location channel searches for objects of interest in the FOV and, after one is found, the classification channel classifies it.

The block diagram follows from biology (figure 5.6). The following paragraphs describe the functions of each module.

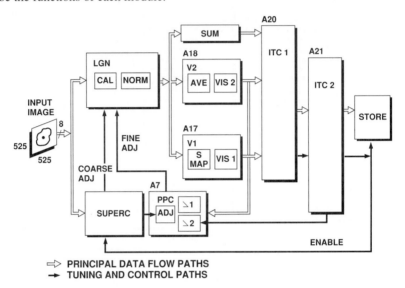

Figure 5.6   Block diagram of a neural network architecture for machine vision. A 525 × 525-pixel image with 8-bit pixels has been included at the left of the figure as an example input image.

To illustrate how the system works, the description carries through an example of a 525 × 525-pixel input image with 8-bit pixels. The example assumes objects of size 175 × 175 pixels appear in the input image. This object size corresponds to normal cells in a Pap smear image at ×400 magnification, discussed below.

1. Classification Channel. Some classification channel modules approximate the functioning of selected brain areas: the lateral geniculate nucleus (LGN), visual area 1 (V1, also called A17), visual area 2 (V2, also called A18), inferior temporal cortex 1 (ITC1, also called A20), and inferior temporal cortex 2 (ITC2, also called A21). Other modules approximate certain biological functions without the anatomical correspondence, such as the SUM module.

2. LGN—Grayness Processing. Figure 5.7 shows the front-end processing stages in the classification channel. The classification channel has feedforward and feedback signals. Signals flow from the input image through the feature extracting stages to ITC1 input.

The first module in the classification channel is the LGN. The LGN contains the CALIBRATE and NORMALIZATION boxes (figure 5.6).

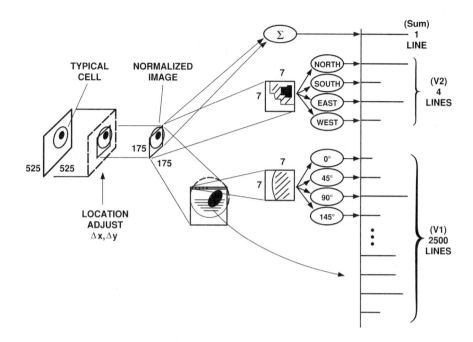

Figure 5.7 Summary of image processing operations. For the example of a 525 × 525-pixel input image, the classification channel places a window of 175 × 175-pixels around the object in the image. (The window size is set to fit the object size.) The 175 × 175 window is then broken into subwindows to extract details of the image, and the details are stored in the feature vector.

The CALIBRATE and NORMALIZATION boxes handle the grayness and adjust for overall illumination in the FOV. These boxes decouple the image's grayness and illumination from the rest of the processing. The decoupling allows designing the remaining modules for pixel values lying in the range of 0 to 1.

Assume the location channel has found an object in the FOV (see below). The location channel sends the pattern's position to the LGN module (figure 5.7, bottom). In the example, the windowed image covers 175 × 175 pixels.

The CALIBRATE box computes a histogram of the windowed image. The testbed images have 8-bit pixels. Histograms of these images are often concentrated in a small band in the range from 0 to 255. Calibrating spreads the intensity values over the entire 0-to-255 range by linearly mapping the lower part to 0 and the upper part to 255.

The histogram's lower limit is the point where the cumulative count is 1 percent of the peak value. The upper limit is where the cumulative count exceeds 99.25 percent. These limits prevent outlying pixel values from affecting the histogram stretching factors.

The NORMALIZE box rescales the pixel values so that pixels leaving the LGN module are in the range from 0 to 1. The box divides the calibrated pixel values by 255.

3. V1—High Resolution Features. The first feature-generating module is A17 (or V1). It breaks the input window into subwindows of 7 × 7 pixels. Thus, the example

175×175-pixel window has 625 subwindows. Note that the 7×7 subwindow size is independent of the input image size.

SPIRAL MAP and VISAREA1 then process each 7×7 subwindow. SPIRAL MAP (figure 5.6) scans through the subwindows in a spiral pattern. The mapping proceeds left to right across the top row, down the right column, right to left across the bottom row, up the left column, back across the second row, and so on. The scanning ends at the center subwindow. The purpose of the spiral mapping is to simplify interpretation of the feature data.

VISAREA1 (figure 5.6) does the high-resolution feature extraction. It measures luminance gradients (increasing or decreasing) in four directions for each 7×7-pixel subwindow.

A gradient is a characteristic of gray images and is analogous to an edge in a binary image. The luminance gradient in the system is the rate of change, or slope, in brightness across a 7×7 subwindow.

Windows with an abrupt step in brightness in one direction have a large gradient in that direction. Windows with a gradual change in brightness from one side to the other have a small gradient. Windows with uniform brightness, that is, with no visible edges, have zero gradient.

The gradients usually differ because the luminance slope depends on direction. The system produces gradients in four directions—vertical, horizontal, and the $45°$ diagonals—for each 7×7 subwindow.

Figure 5.8 shows the operations for producing the four orientation features of each 7×7 subwindow. The system needs only two different NNs, with rotating and reflecting the input.

The gradient detectors in the system are CC NNs. In the testbed, these NNs have 25 hidden neurons and 1 output neuron. As suggested by biology [21], each neuron is excitatory or inhibitory, not both. Figure 5.9 illustrates this NN.

The gradient-measuring NNs give responses to selected patterns. Figure 5.10 shows the design patterns. Each feature detector NN has 1924 fixed interconnecting weights for the testbed.

A genetic algorithm technique computed the weights off-line (see chapter 7). The weights are fixed. Figure 5.11 shows the horizontal responses to the design patterns. Figure 5.12 shows the diagonal responses.

4. V2—Shape Features. The second feature-generating module is A18 (or V2). It detects edges near the perimeter of the input window. V2 is also part of the location channel (see below). Its output contains data about an object's general shape.

The AVERAGE box defocuses the image to produce a single 7×7 image, regardless of the size of the input image (figure 5.6). For the 175×175 input example, the defocusing averages over 25×25 input pixels to produce each output pixel. The averaging smears pattern details (details captured by V1), but retains data about the outside edges.

Figure 5.13 illustrates averaging a cell fully in the window (a) and partly in the window (b). As shown, the averaging produces a single smeared 7×7-pixel image of the pattern in the window.

VISAREA2 detects edges near the four sides of the defocused image. In VISAREA2, a 3×7-pixel detector senses the presence of near-horizontal edges at the top and bottom of

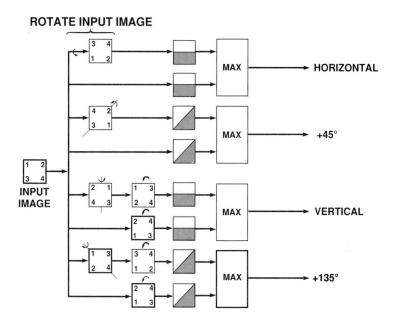

Figure 5.8   Feature detector module for the V1 module. The gray input image is reflected and rotated as shown so that system needs only two neural networks.

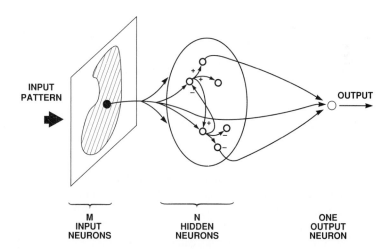

Figure 5.9   Architecture for a feature detector neural network. An input pattern, shown in cross-hatching, is impressed on M neurons. Each input neuron is connected to N hidden neurons and a single output neuron, whose output is high for a chosen angular orientation of the input pattern and low for other orientations. The hidden neurons may be excitatory (labeled $+$) or inhibitory (labeled $-$) and are interconnected. In the baseline system the input pattern is 7×7 pixels with 25 hidden neurons.

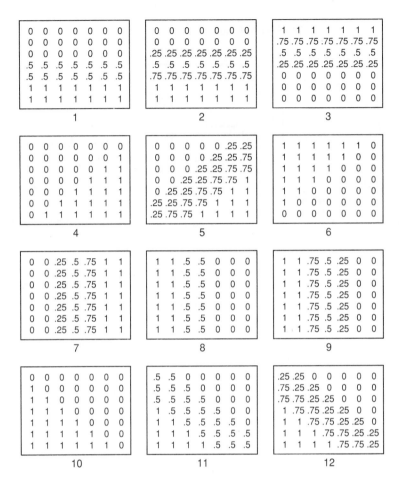

Figure 5.10 Gray patterns used to design the V1 feature detectors, as described in section 7.5. The set includes horizontal (1–3), 45° diagonal (4–6), vertical (7–9), and 135° diagonal (10–12) with two gradient directions.

the smeared image. A 7 × 3-pixel detector senses the presence of near-vertical edges at the right and at the left of the smeared image. Figure 5.14 shows the position of the detectors.

When a window centers on an object, edges occur on four sides. The VISAREA2 output is four values. The values measure the UP, DOWN, RIGHT, and LEFT edge strengths. The feature vector includes these four values, shown in figure 5.15. A single 7 × 3 NN, with rotations and complementing, can do all V2 feature detection.

Figure 5.16 shows the design patterns for VISAREA2. A genetic algorithm technique uses these patterns to design a 7 × 3-pixel input NN (see chapter 7). Patterns 1 to 4 represent edges of a gray image properly windowed. Patterns 5 to 8 represent patterns not properly windowed.

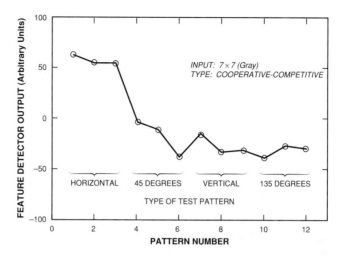

Figure 5.11   Response of the horizontal feature detector to the design patterns.

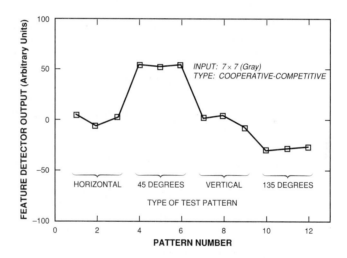

Figure 5.12   Response of the 45° diagonal feature detector to the design patterns.

The VISAREA2 edge detectors use fixed weight CC NNs with 25 neurons and one output. Figure 5.17 shows the response of the V2 vertical (LEFT) edge detector module to the design patterns. The presence of an edge in this section of the image (patterns 1 to 4) gives a large response, while the others (patterns 5 to 8) give small responses.

5. <u>SUM—Size Feature.</u> The third feature-generating module is SUM (figure 5.6). It adds up the pixel values of the input window. Thus, the single output from SUM measures the object's gross size after normalization. For convenience, the architecture separates this

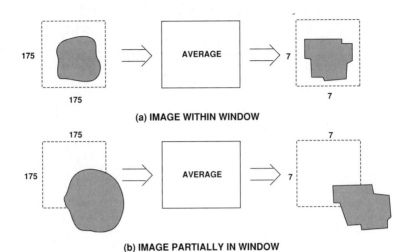

Figure 5.13 The AVERAGE module in V2 takes a, say, 175 × 175-pixel input image and smears its details to give a 7 × 7-pixel output image that retains the general shape information. The position of the input image may be within (a) or outside (b) the window. This position corresponds to the position of the smeared output image.

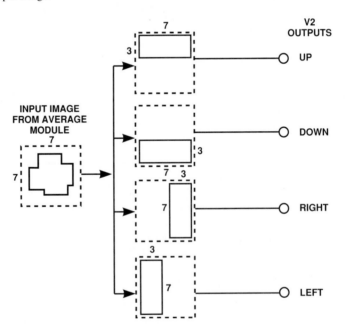

Figure 5.14 Block diagram of the V2 VISAREA2 modules. The modules detect the edges (if any) in 3 × 7- and 7 × 3-pixel sections of the 7 × 7 input image. The four outputs show the presence or absence of an edge in the corresponding section of the 7 × 7 input image.

Another problem associated with current activities on the theory of machine vision is an underlying assumption that a theory of "general" machine vision is achievable. This assumption may be false. [78, p. 189-90]

... standard vision techniques for feature detection, segmentation, recovery, etc., often do not perform very well when applied to natural scenes. [78, p. 867]

Ideally, the [vision process] stages should be closely integrated; the results obtained at a given stage should provide feedback to modify the techniques used at previous stages. This is rarely done in existing vision systems, and as a result, little is known about how to design systems that incorporate feedback between stages. [78, p. 868]

Little is known about visual knowledge representation or about flexible control structures for vision systems. [78, p. 868]

... humans can recognize objects—even complex objects whose presence was unexpected—in a fraction of a second, which is enough time for only a few hundred (!) "cycles" of the neural 'hardware' in the human visual system. Computer vision systems have a long way to go before they will be able to match this performance. [78, p. 868]

In summary, current MV performance is significantly less than the performance of biological vision. Note the references to parallel types of architectures, feedback to earlier stages, and flexible control structures. Note also the need for well-defined problems, a general structure, and applications to natural scenes. The NN architecture described in the preceding section has these features.

SUGGESTED REFERENCES

D. HUBEL, *Eye, Brain, and Vision*. The literature on primate vision is large. Many books deal with this subject alone, and every general treatise on human biology devotes some space to it. Technical journals publish a continuing series of articles on vision. One of the best summaries of this field is by Hubel. It covers the pioneering work of Hubel and Wiesel, whose discoveries have rightly become recognized as of great importance. Although many other works are for the specialist, Hubel's work is pleasantly discursive. His style is less formal and more physical, consequently, more intelligible.

D. ROSE AND V. DOBSON (ed.), *Models of the Visual Cortex*. A quarter of a century has passed since the work of Hubel and Wiesel. During that time there has been a profusion of ideas about the exact nature of the underlying mechanisms in the visual cortex. This book presents the ideas and conclusions of 75 of the most prominent theorists in the field. The subject matter is concentrated on area 17. The mathematics is limited to calculus.

J. MAUNSELL, *Physiological Evidence for Two Visual Subsystems*. Many studies describe two distinct kinds of higher functions in the visual system. One function involves primarily shape, color, and pattern. The other function involves motion and spatial relationships. The paper discusses the behavioral, physiological, and anatomical data bearing on these two visual functions. The functions occur in different brain regions. A duality arises in the organization of the earliest stages of the visual system.

D. VAN ESSEN AND J. MAUNSELL, *Hierarchical Organizations and Functional Streams in the Visual Cortex*. Hubel and Wiesel obtained evidence for many sequential stages of information processing along the visual pathway. As researchers studied the visual pathways in greater detail, they found evidence not supporting a strictly serial scheme of organization. In fact, Hubel and Wiesel's own findings—that area 17 projects to several cortical areas—demonstrates parallel outputs from a single area. The article concerns mainly the relationships among visual areas, rather than with their internal circuitry. It presents evidence for at least two major streams of processing as described in the text.

H. LI AND J. KENDER (eds.), *Computer Vision*. This is an overview of conventional machine vision theory and technology, circa 1988. The 13 papers fall in four groups: introductory, theoretic foundations, hardware architectures, and applications. A main result from this overview is that standard vision techniques for feature detection, segmentation, and so on, often do not perform very well when applied to natural scenes. Human beings can recognize objects—even objects whose presence was unexpected—in a fraction of a second. Computer vision systems have a long way to go before they will be able to match this performance.

J. LLOYD, *Thermal Imaging Systems*. Many studies demonstrate that bar chart equivalents are useful in assessing a machine vision system. Section 10.4 of this reference discusses the bar chart equivalent, known as the Johnson criteria, for detecting (object present), recognition (man or woman), and identification (an individual). The Johnson criteria are a well-known way of connecting laboratory measurements to in-the-field performance.

EXERCISES

1. Design a neural network visual system for reading English letters and words. Size the modules. Describe the training and testing.

2. Design a neural network visual system for recognizing common vehicles at a fixed distance away.

3. Describe how to combine the outputs of two different sensors, say, a video camera and an imaging radar, for increase performance. (*Hint*: Combine the feature detector outputs of the two sensors in one fused feature vector.)

6

Hand-Eye Systems

The preceding chapter considered NN machine vision systems. This chapter extends NN vision by combining vision and motor control. Besides being of practical importance, this material introduces NN control system design from a biological viewpoint.

The program for the chapter is twofold. First, it summarizes selected characteristics of biological motor control. Second, it presents two examples of eye-motor systems that model selected properties.

These eye-motor systems apply the elementary modules derived in preceding chapters. Assuming familiarity with previous material, the discussion emphasizes new themes and the added theory.

6.1 OVERVIEW OF HUMAN MOTOR CONTROL

A long series of investigations have shown the design of motor systems in living creatures. This section summarizes motor control in human beings.

Summarizing [9,56,75] researchers classify muscle as smooth or striated. Smooth muscle appears structureless under the microscope. This muscle is primarily concerned with slow contracts in internal organs and is under involuntary control. Striated muscle, appearing filamentous under the microscope, is cardiac or skeletal. Cardiac muscle produces regular, self-sustaining contractions, controlled by nerves and chemical hormones.

Skeletal muscle—the subject of this chapter—is under voluntary control. Though served by nerves and hormones, the control mechanisms—described below—differ from those of cardiac muscle.

Most striated muscles connect two bones across a joint. (The exceptions are extraocular muscles which move the eyeballs and lingual muscles which move the tongue.) Another muscle opposes every muscle pulling a bone in one direction. That is, there are antagonistic muscle pairs.

Skeletal muscles work in groups. About 650 muscles sheath the human skeleton. One walking step uses about 200 muscles. Forty or more muscles lift a leg and move it forward. Strength depends on the fibers in the muscle. The fibers consist of muscle cells.

Striated muscle cells are a few millimeters long. A membrane called the sarcolemma surrounds these cells. In each cell are many rodlike myofibrils, responsible for the contraction.

A myofibril has repeating light-dark regions, causing the striped appearance of the muscle under the microscope. A myofibril consists of thick filaments sliding inside thin filaments. The thick filaments contain myosin; the thin filaments contain actin.

The sliding-filament model explains contraction. In this model the lengths of the thick and thin filaments remain the same and slide past each other. During contraction the cell length may decrease 50 percent.

The molecular mechanism of muscle contraction is an actin-myosin interaction cycle. The energy source is ATP, discussed in chapter 2.

Motor neurons control muscle contraction. The axons of these neurons release acetylcholine, a neurotransmitter, causing contraction. The axons per motor neuron vary from three for eyeball muscles to hundreds for, say, thigh muscles. Generally, if a single motor neuron innervates few muscle fibers, the movements produced are subtler and more finely graded.

Besides motor neurons, sensory receptors in the muscles give tension measurements, and sensory receptors on tendons give joint positions. Tendons are tough inelastic tissue connecting muscle to bone.

Voluntary movements start in the motor cortex. Like the sensory cortex, the motor cortex has a vertical, columnar organization. Each motor column is a small group of neurons affecting the muscles of a joint. Research shows that movement commands encode to reach a certain joint position, not to activate a series of muscles.

The motor cortex neurons, called Betz cells, communicate directly with the motor neurons of the spinal cord. The axons converge in a large bundle called the pyramidal tract.

Besides the motor cortex, two other brain structures regulate voluntary movements. The basal ganglia in the midbrain, consisting of the striatum, pallidum, subthalamic nucleus, and substantia nigra, gets sensory inputs and starts slow directed large movements. That is, it does coarse adjustments.

The cerebellum in the hindbrain also gets sensory inputs and initiates fast smaller movements. That is, it does fine adjustments. The pyramidal tract sends these adjustments. The cerebellum stores programs of learned movements which the motor cortex can activate.

To make fine adjustments, the cerebellum tracks the position of head and trunk by signals from the muscles and tendons. Large cerebellum neurons called Purkinje cells combine this information, constantly monitoring a map of body position and location. Each Purkinje cell typically gets up to 100,000 inputs from sensory neurons.

6.2 ADAPTIVE EYE-HAND COORDINATION

Developing NN models of the human motor control system is just starting—a task to continue for many years because of its complexity. To date researchers have designed NNs capturing some important biological characteristics. And indeed, practical applications of these control systems are also starting.

This section and the next describe example NN eye-motor control systems inspired by biology. These systems develop accurate sensory-motor coordination despite changes in the body dimensions, motor strength, and unpredictable events. Moreover, this coordination is automatic.

For simplicity consider a system consisting of two eyes and one arm. The purpose of the system is to look at an object and reach for it with the arm. The system trains and corrects itself. (The model can easily be generalized to more sensory inputs and more limb joints.)

Following Kuperstein [57], develop the system as follows:

1. Arm-Muscle Signals. Assume a limb consisting of two joints, a shoulder, and an elbow. To introduce notation, let a_{pq} be the arm-muscle signals, shown in figure 6.1.

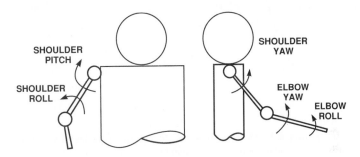

Figure 6.1 Nomenclature for a simple two-joint limb. Arm-muscle signals, a_{pq}, activate antagonistic muscle pairs ($p = 1, 2$) in five degrees of freedom ($q = 1, \ldots, 5$). For the shoulder, $q = 1$ (roll), $q = 2$ (pitch), and $q = 3$ (yaw). For the elbow, $q = 4$ (roll) and $q = 5$ (yaw).

Denote the antagonistic muscle pairs by $p = 1, 2$. Denote shoulder roll, pitch, and yaw by $q = 1, 2$, and 3. Denote elbow roll by $q = 4$ and yaw by $q = 5$.

2. Joint-Angle Activation. Assume a joint angle is linearly proportional to the muscle activation. Assume a monotonic dependency between angle and activation (this is a major assumption—see section 6.3).

3. Eye-Muscle Signals. The signals that contract and point each eye are e_{pq}. Denote the antagonistic muscle pairs by $p = 1, 2$. Following human biology, an eye is pulled in three directions spaced 60° apart. The direction indices are $q = 1, 2$, and 3 (figure 6.2). Denote the right-eye signals by e^r_{pq} and the left-eye signals by e^l_{pq}.

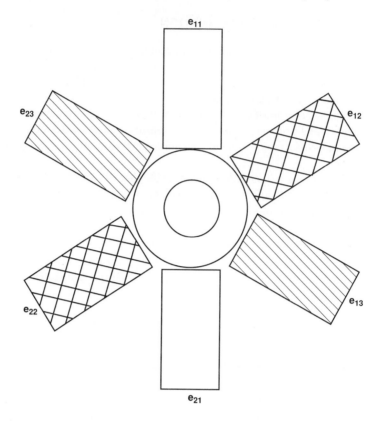

Figure 6.2   Nomenclature for the eye-ball muscles. Eye-muscle signals, e_{pq}, activate antagonistic muscle pairs ($p = 1, 2$) in three directions spaced $60°$ apart ($q = 1, 2, 3$).

4. Retinal Map. Each eye registers light intensity on a two-dimensional space. The light intensity at position i, j is v_{ij}. Denote the right eye by v_{ij}^r and the left eye by v_{ij}^l. The indices $i = 1, 2, \ldots, I$ and $j = 1, 2, \ldots, J$ span the two-dimensional visual space.

5. Eye Foveation. This system relates e_{pg} and v_{ij} of each eye. Many models are possible. For simplicity, assume the system points the eyeballs toward the visual center of an object in the field of view, shown in figure 6.3. (For a better model use the material on vision in chapter 5.)

6. Gaze Map. Biology vision systems do not have sensors directly measuring eye position, so the eye position must be computed from the eye signals. The gaze map gives the eye positions from the foveation signals.

The gaze map is three distributions of activations, $E_{pq<i>}^r$, $E_{pq<i>}^l$, and $E_{pq<i>}^d$, which give right, left, and difference (disparity) in eye pointing.

The recruitment function gives the gaze map as follows:

$$E_{pq<i>} = \{f(i)[e_{pq} - g(i)]\}^+, \tag{6.1}$$

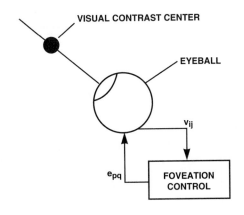

Figure 6.3 Foveation system for pointing a sensor. An eye foveation control system points the two eyes toward the visual contrast center of an object in the visual field of view.

where

$$f(i) = \alpha \frac{i}{I}, \ i = 1, \ldots, I \tag{6.2}$$

and

$$g(i) = \beta \frac{i}{I}, \ i = 1, \ldots, I. \tag{6.3}$$

These equations model the oculomotor nuclei in the midbrain, shown schematically in figure 6.4.

7. Retinal and Orientation Maps. In human beings the visual cortex processes retinal maps for orientations in lines, slots, and edges. The result of this processing is the orientation maps.

To model visual cortex processing, assume the system is sensitive to orientations in four directions: $0°$, $45°$, $90°$, and $135°$. Assume a convolution gives this processing, as follows.

$$V_{x<ij>} = v_{<ij>} * k_x, \tag{6.4}$$

where k_x are kernel matrices.

The kernel matrices have the same negative coefficients everywhere except along one string in one of four orientations. The coefficients in that string are the same positive number.

Comparing $V_{x<ij>}^r$ and $V_{x<ij>}^l$ gives $V_{x<ij>}^d$. Interleave the $V_{x<ij>}$ elements to form the visual map. The visual map mimics the retinotopic layout of neural responses in the A-17 visual cortex, shown in figure 6.5. (See chapter 5 for a better model of the feature detectors.)

8. Weight Maps. Combine the gaze and visual maps through weight maps to produce arm-muscle signals. Let $W_{ij<pq>}$ be weight maps used to gate (multiply) the gaze map and the visual map. The ij indices give the map position in the two-dimensional gaze map and the visual map. The pq indices give the limb-muscle elements.

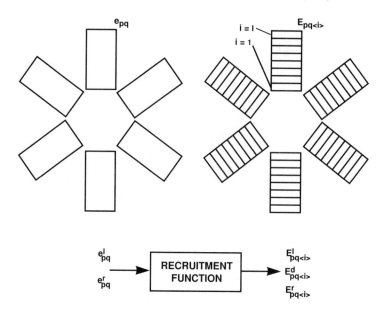

Figure 6.4   Gaze map schematic. The gaze map is a set of three neural activations $E^l_{pq<i>}$ (left), $E^r_{pq<i>}$ (right), and $E^d_{pq<i>}$ (disparity), where p, q are as
in figure 6.3 and $i = 1, \ldots, I$ (network population). The recruitment function
maps the eye-muscle signals to the three activation distributions. The gaze map
mimics neural responses in the oculomotor nuclei of the midbrain.

9. Motor Signals. Assume computed motor signals, from gaze and vision, are M'_{pq}.
Compute $\overline{M'_{pq}}$ by

$$M'_{pq} = \sum_{i,j} S_{ij} W_{ij<pq>}, \tag{6.5}$$

where S_{ij} is an element from the gaze map or the visual map.

10. Arm-Muscle Signals. The motor signals from the brain produce the arm-muscle
signals. Assume

$$a_{pq} = \frac{M_{pq} + M'_{pq}}{\sum_p (M_{pq} + M'_{pq})}, \tag{6.6}$$

where M_{pq} is the actual motor signal traveling from brain to spinal cord. At first, the arm-
muscle signals may be random. Note, the denominator normalizes the antagonistic muscle
pairs.

11. Learning Rule. Learning adjusts the weight maps of the system. Comparing the
actual and computed motor signals produces an error, which is

$$\epsilon_{pq} = M_{pq} - M'_{pq}. \tag{6.7}$$

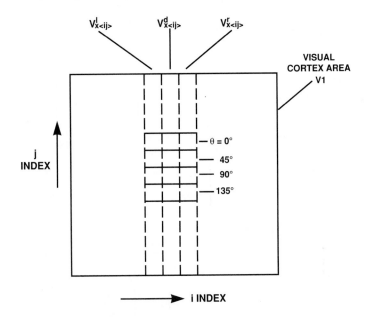

Figure 6.5   Visual map schematic. The visual map is a set of neural activations $V^l_{x<ij>}$ (left), $V^r_{x<ij>}$ (right), and $V^d_{x<ij>}$ (disparity), where $< ij >$ are the two-dimensional coordinates of the retina and x indexes the orientation, say, $0°$, $45°$, $90°$, and $135°$. The visual map mimics the retinotopic layout of some neural responses in the visual cortex.

The learning rule

$$W (n + 1)_{ij<pq>} = W (n)_{ij<pq>} + \sigma S_{ij} \epsilon_{pq} \qquad (6.8)$$

adjusts the weight maps, where σ is the learning rate.

Figure 6.6 shows a block diagram of the system. The system is first trained and then operated as follows.

12. Training Procedure. To train the system, follow these steps:

a. Initialize $W_{ij<qp>} = 0$.

b. Choose random values for the motor signals, M_{pq}, and for the object positions in the FOV.

c. Foveate on the object.

d. Compute the gaze map and the visual map.

e. Update the weight map by the learning rule.

f. Repeat steps (b) to (e) for other motor signals and other object positions.

13. Operating. After training, the system can accurately reach for objects. First, the eyes search and find an object in the FOV. Second, the system computes motor signals. Third, the signals move the limb to reach the object.

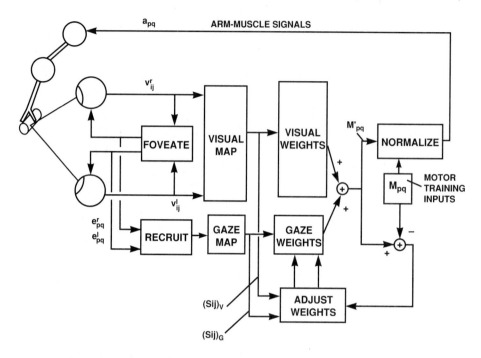

Figure 6.6   Block diagram of a neural network for adaptive hand-eye coordination. During learning, a random generator produces signals positioning the arm while the hand holds an object. The two eyes orient to the object. The eye-muscle signals transform to a gaze map. The visual signals transform to a visual map. Stereo views of the object register in the retinas. The V1 module processes these images for orientation and disparity. The visual weights gate signals from each visual map unit to each arm-muscle unit. Normalizing the sum of the products of gaze map and visual map produces the arm-muscle signals. The comparator matches these gaze-visual product signals. The difference changes the values in the two weight maps.

During learning, a random generator produces signals positioning the arm while the hand holds an object. The two eyes orient to the object.

The eye-muscle signals transform to a gaze map. Each leg of the gaze map represents the pulling direction of either eye. The gaze-map values (weights) gate signals from each gaze map unit to each arm-muscle unit.

The visual signals transform to a visual map. First, stereo views of the object register in the retinas. In each trial, the V1 module processes these images for orientation and disparity. The visual map interleaves the orientation and disparity responses from the two eyes. The visual weights gate signals from each visual map unit to each arm-muscle unit.

Normalizing the sum of the products of gaze map and visual map produces the arm-muscle signals. The comparator matches these gaze-visual product signals. The difference changes the values in the two weight maps.

Common simplifying assumptions include arranging the neurons in layers, no lateral connections in a layer, and only feedforward signals between layers. Or, a neuron can be both excitatory and inhibitory. That is, the connection weights from a neuron to others, modeling synaptic transmission coupling, can be positive to some and negative to others.

These assumptions are significant restrictions, especially in modeling biological systems. Moreover, they differ from our present knowledge of the anatomy and physiology of the cerebral cortex of higher animals [21].

Nevertheless, with these assumptions, researchers have developed design methods for many kinds of NNs. For NN feature detectors, a common design is to compute the output by convolving the input pattern with a kernel matrix. The designer selects the kernel matrix so that the output measures, say, the orientation of an edge in the input pattern. The response mimics the orientation responses to illumination contrast of simple cells in the visual cortex [51].

While mathematically convenient, the method is at best a rough approximation of biological feature detectors because convolution is linear. Nonlinear feature detectors may be better, although no careful study is known to the author. Indeed, designing these nonlinear NNs is difficult. A typical robotic application with this design is by Kuperstein [57], discussed in chapter 6.

In feedforward NNs, adjusting connection weights is currently done by the simulated annealing (SA) and backpropagation (BP) methods. SA includes the Boltzmann machine [1] and is slow. BP is the most common method. Werbos [84] originated BP, and Rumelhart (1986) and other members of the PDP group [79] developed it.

Though advances continue, nevertheless, BP—and its many variations—suffer from slowness for many problems [44], besides being restricted to feedforward NNs.

Adaptive Resonance Theory (ART) architectures, discussed in chapter 4, are NNs that usually function with variable—not fixed—interconnections among the neurons. Designing ART NNs is not considered here [14,15,16].

Many applications have assemblies of fixed and variable modules, as shown in chapters 5 and 6. The variable modules, those with learning, may use an ART NN. The fixed modules—say the feature detectors—may use a NN designed by the technique described below. Thus, the NNs with fixed interconnections are important in modeling and applications.

The GA design method described below does not make the common assumptions. Thus, it should be of interest to theorists and to designers of applications. Indeed, the resulting NNs may be smaller for the same function and easier to implement in software or hardware.

7.2 GENETIC ALGORITHM BACKGROUND

For over a decade the GA community, originated by Holland [48], has pursued trial-and-error strategies for designing adaptive systems. The GA is a search procedure, inspired by evolution and heredity, for finding high performance structures in a complex parameter domain.

For NN design purposes, the GA is a search method for finding a good set of weights in a high-dimensional nonlinear weight space. (Degenerate forms of the GA are the well-known gradient-descent techniques, including BP.)

Holland originated two distinct GA approaches. Researchers named the two approaches—Michigan and Pittsburgh—after the communities where they were first elaborated.

In the Michigan approach a single system consists of a set of rules, or parameters. Genetic operators applied to existing rules discover new rules. The approach assigns a value to each rule, expressing the rule's fitness for reaching a payoff. Rules earn high value by achieving direct payoff in the task environment, or by setting the stage for later rules.

Thus, in the Michigan approach, the GA operates on the rules—or internal parameters—of a single system. The GA picks the "best rules" as the system adapts to an environment.

In the Pittsburgh approach many systems, each with a set of rules, compete. Holland's original book defined reproductive plans [48, pp. 90–111]. A reproductive plan maintains a set of possible systems. The plan selects an individual system according to its performance rank, modifies it by one or more genetic operators, evaluates it by the environment that contains external inputs, and then replaces a randomly selected member of the set by it.

In the Pittsburgh approach the set of systems evolves to contain members with high performance, because the better an individual performs, the more offspring it has.

The Michigan approach is most practical in on-line real-time environments because of the reduced computational loads. The Pittsburgh approach is appropriate in off-line environments where more leisurely exploration is acceptable.

In GA terminology, this chapter uses primarily a Michigan approach.

GA theory gives guidelines for constructing practical search techniques [7,25]. (A direct random search of parameter space is not practical because the trials increase exponentially with the neurons.)

The fundamental requirements are that the problem be represented by some data structure, the solutions be capable of evaluation, the advances already made be retained, and the population of retained structures be increased.

In GA applications the major problems are finding a convenient representation of the system, devising genetic operators that produce good solutions, and defining payoff functions.

Following these guidelines, define a GA as follows. First, create a set of structures—generation—that try to solve a problem. Second, manipulate the structures—parents—by a set of genetic operators (traditionally crossover, inversion, and mutation) to create a new set of structures. Third, evaluate the new structures on how well they solve the problem. Fourth, save the best set of structures—the next generation. Fifth, repeat the process until a structure produces an acceptable solution to the problem.

Researchers have applied the GA to design simple NNs. Recent examples are Miller, Todd, and Hegde [68], who assume a feedforward NN. A matrix of digits denotes the nature of interconnections among the neurons. The GA picks rows of this matrix and swaps with the parent. The resulting NN is trained by BP and evaluated.

Whitley and Hansen [85] represent a feedforward NN in binary form with 4 or 8 bits for each connecting weight. They concatenate the weight bits to form a string, which an adaptive mutation operator manipulates. They then train the NN by BP and evaluate it.

Harp, Samad, and Guha [37] also represent connections by a bit string, use the standard mutation operator, and train the system by BP. Their studies, considering only simple examples like the XOR problem, assume feedforward NNs, BP-related performance metrics, and binary string representations for the connection weights.

Cellier [19], in a chapter entitled "Artificial NNs and Genetic Algorithms," describes a GA method that defines four classes of values for the weights ranging from very small to very large. He assigns each weight to a size class and arranges the size labels (A, B, C, D) in a string, for example, ABACCBDADBCBBADCA. The number of labels is the number of weights. The method generates a hundred strings to form a genetic pool. Then he applies the crossover and mutation GA operators to produce new strings that they evaluate and sort. He applies this GA method to design feedforward NNs with 67 unknown parameters.

The remainder of this chapter describes a method for designing NNs with fixed connection weights. It demonstrates the method by nontrivial examples—75 neurons, 1920 connection weights—of orientation detectors modeling simple cell modules in the visual cortex of primates. Moreover, the design examples satisfy important biological constraints.

7.3 FORMULATION

1. Activation Equation. Suppose a set of neurons $\{v_i\}$ form a feature detector module. Describe each neuron by equations that roughly model the biological processes. Following chapter 2, characterize the ith neuron, v_i, by its activation level, x_i, and by its connections with other neurons. Give the connections by a set of coupling coefficients, $\{Z_{ji}\}$.

For the activation level, or short-term memory (STM), assume an equation for v_i of the form

$$\frac{dx_i}{dt} = -\alpha x_i + \sum_j Z_{ji} f(x_j) + I_i, \; \forall i, \qquad (7.1)$$

where

$$
\begin{aligned}
x_i &= \text{activation of the } i\text{th neuron,} \\
Z_{ji} &= \text{long-term memory (LTM) trace from the } j\text{th neuron to the } i\text{th neuron,} \\
I_i &= \text{external input to the } i\text{th neuron,} \\
f(\ ) &= \text{a nonlinear signal function,} \\
\alpha &= \text{relaxation time constant parameter.}
\end{aligned}
$$

This equation, called the additive STM equation, is basic in NN research and is adequate for many NN designs. (If desired, replace the additive STM equation by the shunting STM equation for a better model of the biology—see chapter 2).

Assume the coupling coefficients (or the LTM traces) are constant and unknown.

For this class of NNs with fixed interconnections, the main problem is to find a set of weights, $\{Z_{ji}\}$, satisfying prescribed I/O relations.

To illustrate the method, the following discussion considers a feature detector module. Designing NNs for other functions using a similar method follows.

A simple design of a feature detector module gives a single output for some spatial activation pattern defined on an array of input neurons. The output could show the, say, angular orientation of the pattern.

For a feature detector assume input patterns defined on M input neurons, N hidden (internal) neurons, and a single output neuron. Thus, each input pattern is characterized by the activation level of a single output neuron, as shown in chapter 5, figure 5.9.

The input pattern may be binary or gray, that is, the inputs, I_i, may have values 0 or 1 (binary) or, say, 0, 1, 2, ..., 255 (7 bits of gray).

Assume no feedback from the hidden neurons or from the output neuron to the input neurons. Nevertheless, assume feedback among the hidden neurons and assume direct connections from the input neurons to the output neuron.

For this example, write a set of STM equations from (7.1) as follows.

- Input Neurons

$$\frac{dx_i}{dt} = -\alpha x_i + I_i, \ i = 1, \ldots, M. \tag{7.2}$$

- Hidden Neurons

$$\frac{dx_i}{dt} = -\alpha x_i + \sum_{j=1}^{M+N} Z_{ji} f(x_j), \ i = 1, \ldots, N. \tag{7.3}$$

- Output Neuron

$$\frac{dx_0}{dt} = -\alpha x_0 + \sum_{j=1}^{M+N} Z_{j0} f(x_j). \tag{7.4}$$

2. Matrix Formulation. Write the STM equations of the hidden neurons as

$$\frac{dx_i}{dt} = -\alpha x_i + \sum_{j=1}^{N} Z_{ji} f(x_j) + \sum_{k=1}^{M} Z'_{ki} f(x_k), \ i = 1, \ldots, N, \tag{7.5}$$

where

Z_{ji} = LTM trace of the hidden neurons,

Z'_{ki} = LTM trace from the input neurons to the hidden neurons.

Assume $\alpha = 1$ (equivalent to rescaling the other variables). Then, the input neuron activations approach the external inputs, that is, $x_k \rightarrow I_k, k = 1, \ldots, M$ as $t \rightarrow \infty$ in the steady state. Assume no self-sustained oscillations.

In the steady state the hidden neuron activations become

$$x_i = \sum_{j=1}^{N} Z_{ji} f(x_j) + \sum_{k=1}^{M} Z'_{ki} f(I_k), \ i = 1, \ldots, N. \tag{7.6}$$

Table 7.1 shows the assumed parameters for the GA design example. The example assumes an input pattern defined on 7×7 or 49 input neurons. (A NN with an angular resolution of, say, $10°$ would have more input neurons and could also be designed by this method.) The hidden system has 25 neurons.

TABLE 7.1. INPUT PARAMETERS FOR DESIGNING A HORIZONTAL FEATURE DETECTOR USING AN ON-CENTER-OFF-SURROUND NEURAL NETWORK

Input neurons (M)	7×7 (49)
Hidden neurons (N)	25
Copies per generation	10
Fraction of weights changed	
Per copy	1/3
Search range	$0, \pm 1, \pm 2, \ldots, \pm 10$
High band	50 to 100
Low band	-100 to 10

Starting with a random set $\{\mathbf{A}, \mathbf{B}, \mathbf{C}, \mathbf{D}\}$ for the first generation, at each generation ten copies are made of the parent set.

For each copy, a third of the matrix elements (weights) are randomly changed by selecting integer values over the range -10 to $+10$, subject to the constraints given in section 7.3.

Assume a HI-LO metric for the training patterns with some of the outputs in a high band and the others in a low band. That is, the desired output response to the high (horizontal) training patterns is 50 to 100. The desired response to the low (nonhorizontal) training patterns is -100 to 10.

Row-by-row scanning produces the input vector, $\mathbf{I}$, for each training pattern. That is, I_1 to I_7 are the first row, I_8 to I_{14} are the second row, and I_{43} to I_{49} are the seventh row. The example determines 1924 coefficients for this NN. For simplicity, assume the signal function is a unit step.

Compute the HI-LO metrics of the ten copies and compare them with the metric of the parent set. If an offspring metric is below the parent metric, the offspring replaces the parent set for the next generation.

Figure 7.3 shows 12 training patterns. For a horizontal detector assume the desired responses are high (50 to 100) to the horizontal patterns and are low (-100 to 10) to the others. As seen, training is on three horizontal patterns and nine other patterns. Each training pattern has about two hidden neurons.

The design algorithm was coded in the APL*PLUS programming language and run on an 8-MHz IBM PC/AT machine. Figure 7.4 shows the history of the metric as the system evolves to a solution in about 600 generations. The metric started at $d = 10$ and ended at $d = 1$ at 600 generations. The one remaining error was a response above the high threshold, and so the run was stopped.

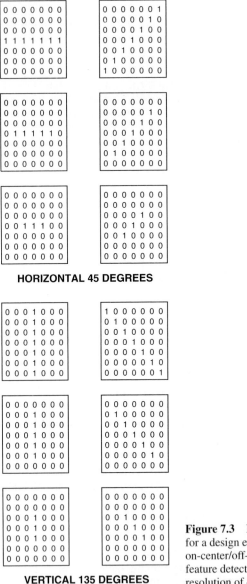

HORIZONTAL 45 DEGREES

VERTICAL 135 DEGREES

Figure 7.3 Binary training patterns for a design example of an on-center/off-surround architecture feature detector with an angular resolution of 45°.

Figure 7.5 shows the resulting system's response to the training patterns. It shows that the high-to-low responses—the signal-to-noise ratio—is above 5, corresponding to the responses of horizontal-to-nonhorizontal training patterns.

The second design example is an ON CTR/OFF SUR NN sensitive to 45° binary patterns on a square array of neurons with a resolution of 45°. All parameters are the same as in the horizontal example. The payoff criterion is different.

For this NN, the high responses are the 45° training patterns, and the others have a low response.

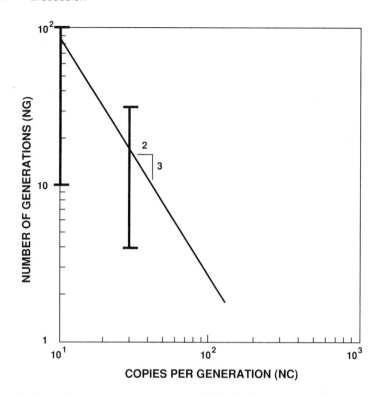

Figure 7.8   Scaling for the design generations versus the copies made each generation for cooperative-competitive architectures. The brackets show the range of the design examples.

7.7 DISCUSSION

This chapter gives a unified, practical method for designing complex, fixed interconnected NNs that realizes designer-specified I/O characteristics and (if desired) meets constraints emerging from the experimental studies of natural brains. By a GA, the chapter gives a convenient representation, a genetic operator, and a payoff function.

The chapter also describes designing CC and ON CTR/OFF SUR NNs that model orientation detectors in the visual cortex and that meet specified I/O functions according to two criteria. Moreover, examples show the method produces NN designs with good output signal-to-noise margins. Finally, some rough guidelines for selecting parameters are given for CC NNs.

The method has several extensions of interest to theorists and application designers. In the applications, designers can apply the technique to multiple-output NNs with specified I/O properties. Designs have been done of NNs with two outputs for a control system (see problems). For the theorists, researchers can model veto cells and neural systems with diffuse inputs, described in Crick and Asanama [21].

While this chapter describes a few examples, and those not thoroughly, nevertheless, the sheer simplicity and flexibility of the method suggest further study is worthwhile.

SUGGESTED REFERENCES

J. HOLLAND, *Adaptation in Natural and Artificial Systems*. The literature on the genetic algorithm is extensive. One of the best is the original work by Holland. The work contains much material not readily available elsewhere. Discussions of the underlying concepts are long and elaborate. It lays the foundations of the Michigan and Pittsburgh approaches.

Proceedings of International Conference on Genetic Algorithms and Their Applications. This conference series illustrates applying GA to many fields, including NNs. The series is recommended for background.

G. ADOMIAN AND G. E. ADOMIAN, *A Global Method for Solution of Complex Systems*. This is a tutorial paper introducing a method for solving dynamic systems that may be strongly nonlinear. The method is applicable to a wide class of problems in physics, engineering, and other disciplines.

EXERCISES

1. Starting with the text design method, describe a NN design technique for M-inputs, two-outputs. Include a description of the payoff criterion.

2. Assume designs of NN edge detectors have been found for $0°$ and $45°$ (see text examples). Using these NN modules, develop a block diagram for feature detector modules that have an angular resolution of $45°$. That is, they measure the edge strength of input patterns at angles $0°$, $45°$, $90°$, and $135°$. (*Hint*: Rotate the input patterns.)

8

Brain Control
and Modulation Systems

NN theory is contributing to understanding normal and abnormal behavior in human beings. The advantages of the NN approach lie in its deeper insights, primarily from the ideas of pattern mixing, matching, stability, switching, and enhancement. As a result, we are led to a new view of mental functioning. This chapter presents an overview of global brain-mind functioning and relates it to NNs.

The NN viewpoint is also of interest for constructing theories of complex processing and for being potentially of considerable help in treating mental illness. Indeed, a NN theory of human behavior serves as a point of departure for theories about complex networks. The equal status accorded to thought and neuron-activation patterns suggests designing machines that think and understand.

8.1 INTRODUCTION

Researchers have produced hypotheses connecting NNs and human brain-mind functioning, all having some experimental support. First, all mental functioning is pattern processing by neuron activity. This includes perception, emotion, cognition, learning, memory, and motor control.

Second, a central control system coordinates the pattern processing in different brain modules. Monamine neurotransmitters, primarily, exert control chemically. In each brain module the monamine neurotransmitters perform many functions. They regulate pattern formation, stabilize node encoding, mix sensory inputs, and match short-term and long-term memory traces.

Third, mental disorders, such as manic-depression and schizophrenia, are malfunctions of the control system. Thus, mental disorders are breakdowns in pattern processing. Indeed, a task just starting connects a mental illness to a pattern processing dysfunction and then to a control system malfunction.

Fourth, NN theory describes pattern development and processing in human beings.

Thus, NNs, control theory, and physiology together increase the understanding of human behavior and psychology.

The next sections develop these hypotheses.

8.2 NEUROTRANSMITTERS

A basic issue in neuroscience is how the brain-mind represents information. The NN answer is that patterns of neural activity—established by LTM traces—represent information. Neurotransmitters in the synapses produce the LTM traces.

(Current NN theory may be expanded to include new results in cellular and molecular biology summarized by Black [8]. The NN models discussed in this text are a first approximation to better models—see section 2.4.)

The traditional biochemical view of the synapse considers neurotransmitters for control and for processing. The neurotransmitters for information processing have receptors with fast (1 ms) response times. Those neurotransmitters for control have receptors with slow (100 ms and longer) response times.

The two classes of fast and slow neurotransmitters have other distinguishing characteristics. Table 8.1 shows a classification of neurotransmitters, their effect, and their function. Information processing in the CNS comes from the γ-aminobutyric acid (GABA) or actetylcholine (ACh) neurotransmitters.

TABLE 8.1.   CLASSIFICATION OF NEUROTRANSMITTERS

Response Time	Effect	Drug Class	Principal Molecule	Function
Fast (1 ms)	Excitatory Inhibitory		Glulamate GABA	Information Processing
Slow (100 ms to 100 s)	Excitatory	Neuropeptides Monamines	— DA NA	Control and modulation
	Inhibitory	Neuropeptides Monamines	— 5-HT ACh	

DA = dopamine; NA = norepinephrine; 5-HT = serotonin;
ACh = acetylcholine; GABA = γ-aminobutyric acid.

Control and modulation in the CNS come from amines such as norepinephrine (NA), serotonin (5-HT), and dopamine (DA). They modulate by changing the effects of other neurotransmitters, that is, by making other neurotransmitters less effective, or preventing release altogether.

Indeed, two different neurotransmitters, such as an amine and a peptide, can coexist in the same synapses. Moreover, the mode of action for control can be quite different from the punctual actions of GABA or ACh for processing.

The neurotransmitter release sites may not be close to the postsynaptic membrane. Transmitters may diffuse widely to affect distant targets and thus, influence many neurons rather uniformly. Table 8.2 shows the control and modulation function of common neurotransmitters in mammalian CNS.

TABLE 8.2. SUMMARY OF NEUROTRANSMITTERS FOR
CONTROL AND MODULATION OF THE CENTRAL NERVOUS
SYSTEM

Transmitter	Effect	Source	Target	Action
DA	+	SN	Basal Ganglia	Damage of SN causes movement disorders.
			Cortex	Parkinson's (DA ↓) Schizophrenia (DA ↑)
NA	+	LC	Cerebellar Purkinje cells Cerebral cortex Thalamus	Destruction of LC changes development of visual cortex.
5-HT	−	RN	Ubiquitous No synaptic specialization	Level of wakefulness Pain sensation

DA = dopamine; NA = norepinephrine; 5-HT = serotonin;
SN = substantia nigra; LC = locus coeruleus; RN = raphe nuclei;
(+) = excitatory; (-) = inhibitory.

Figure 8.1 shows the molecular structure of common neurotransmitters. Biogenic amines, that is, those needed for the life process, include 5-HT, NA, DA, and epinephrine (EP). Of these amines, the catecholamines contain a benzene ring with two adjacent hydroxyl groups.

Enzymes synthesize the catechols from dietary tyrosine in the following sequence: tyrosine → L-Dopa → DA → NA → EP [8, p. 27].

A common feature of mammalian brains is discrete neurons groups sharing the same neurotransmitter. Thus, populations of neurons containing 5-HT, NA, and DA aggregate in separate clusters.

Small groups of nerve cells in discrete locations in the CNS are the principal—and sometimes the only—sources of axons containing 5-HT, DA, and NA. The axons branch extensively to supply widespread areas of the brain, with profound consequences.

Synapses continually secrete neurotransmitters, as described in chapter 2. Indeed, how the brain produces and transports neurotransmitters is an active research area. Neuro-

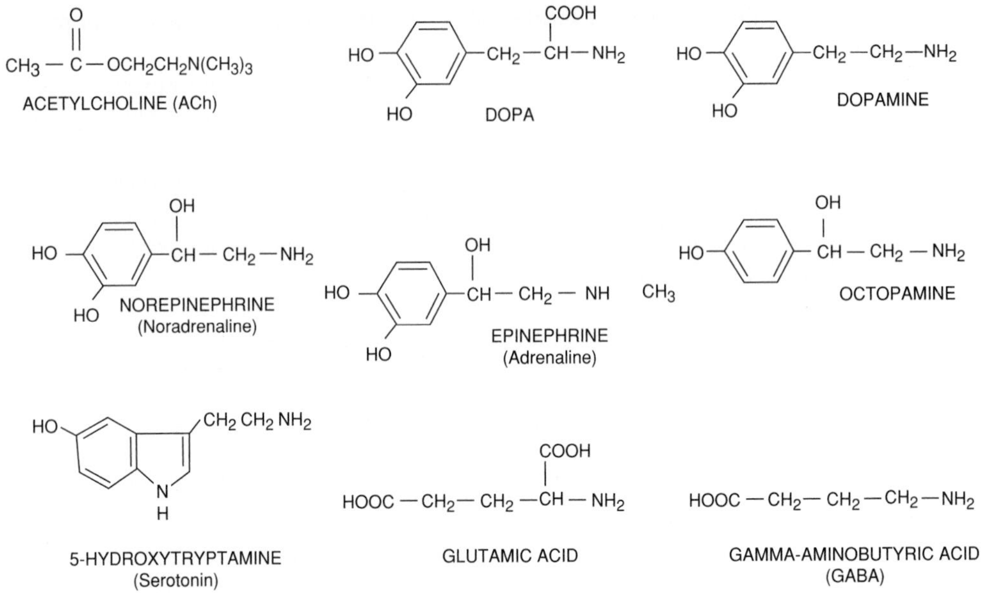

Figure 8.1   Chemical structures of neurotransmitters. (From Kuffler et al. *From Neuron to Brain*. Reprinted by permission of Sinauer Associates, Inc., 1984).

transmitters may be shipped ready-made to the synapses from another site. They may be assembled from parts from the cell body. Or, they may be synthesized at the synapse.

For example, tryptophan—the amino acid precursor of 5-HT—is brought to the presynapic neuron through the blood. 5-HT is synthesized from tryptophan inside the axon terminal and stored in vesicles.

8.3 THE MONAMINE CONTROL SYSTEM

Experiments show that the monamine neurotransmitters control and modulate the activities of different brain modules. Evidence of monamine effects on global mental functions is also well-known.

At least three monamines dominate. They are DA, NA, and 5-HT. DA and NA are excitatory; 5-HT is primarily inhibitory.

Summarizing [46], anatomical evidence in mammals shows a direct pathway from the limbic system through the nucleus accumbeus (NAC) to the pallidum. Researchers believe the pallidum is the motor output for the basal ganglia.

This pathway initiates and executes goal-oriented behavior. For this reason it is called the execution pathway, shown in figure 8.2.

The execution pathway turns impulses produced by the limbic system into motor outputs to the spinal column. The origin of limbic and neocortex outputs in turn involves higher-level processing.

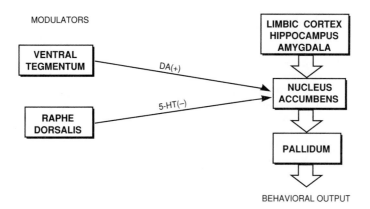

Figure 8.2   Model for the execution pathway producing and controlling behaviors. (From Hestenes. A Neural Network of Theory of Manic-Depressive Illness in Levine and Leven (eds.). *Motivation, Emotion, and Goal Direciton in Neural Networks.* Reprinted with permission of D. Hestenes and Lawrence Erlbaum Associates, Inc., 1992).

Anatomic evidence suggests the NAC is a gate—or switch—through which the limbic system affects behavior. Evidence suggests DA inputs from the ventral tegmentum (VT) open the NAC gate, and 5-HT inputs from the raphe dorsalis (RD) close the NAC gate. The VT and RD are nuclei of neurons in the midbrain and central brainstem.

Thus, the execution pathway starts and actuates goal-directed behavior. Evidence supports the following observations.

Stimulating the NAC with DA agonists (elevators) causes hyperactivity because DA has an excitatory effect facilitating passage of limbic signals. Common DA agonists are amphetamine and cocaine. Stimulating DA antagonists (suppressors) reduce activity.

This evidence leads to the hypothesis that manic-depression (M-D) is caused by malfunctioning VT/DA regulation. That is, patients exhibit manic symptoms—impulsive behavior and pressured speech—because of high DA. They exhibit depressive symptoms—inability to experience pleasure—because of low DA.

In contrast, 5-HT inputs from the RD have an inhibitory effect opposing the facilitatory effect of VT/DA input.

Anatomic evidence also suggests a second parallel pathway. This pathway, called the selection pathway, organizes and selects behavior plans. The selection pathway has direct access to sensory and motor data.

Figure 8.3 shows the selection pathway. The striatum plays the same gating role as the NAC. Moreover, the striatum is controlled like the NAC.

Combining the execution and selection pathways gives the behavioral control system. Figure 8.4 shows the overall functional organization of the system. Although the anatomical components and connections are well known, researchers understand their functions poorly.

Thus, two pathways select and execute behavioral plans. They converge at the pallidum where the final decision is made and broadcast by releasing GO signals (see chapter 6) to the spinal column.

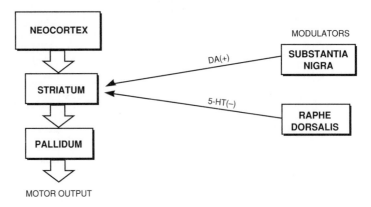

Figure 8.3   Model for the selection pathway organizing and controlling behaviors.

Inhibition control is by 5-HT neurotransmitters of the RM and RD neurons. RM projects to limbic components, while RD projects to motor components in the two pathways.

Excitatory control is by DA neurotransmitters of the VT and SN neurons. VT regulates the execution pathway, and SN regulates the selection pathway. A feedback path, VT → NAC → SN, coordinates the two pathways.

The RD also exerts indirect control by projecting to the VT and SN as well as direct control of the NAC and STR. This control inhibits DA output and is a mechanism for 5-HT simultaneously regulating DA gain in the VT and the SN.

Moreover, the RD responds to stress and to external stimuli. When stress occurs, locus coeruleus (LC) signals inhibit the RD. Thus, stress prepares the NAC, VT, and SN for vigorous behavioral response by increasing DA. Experimentally, RD lesions stop DA responses to stress stimuli.

8.4 CORTICAL CONTROL MODULES

The RD and LC modules play major roles in modulation processing. RD neurons, which innervate the entire neocortex, have a slow regular output. During sleep, RD outputs decrease, going to zero during paradoxical sleep. The effects are slow to start and slow to end. That is, the time constant is long. Moreover, the responses to inputs are nonspecific and stereotyped.

LC neurons also innervate the entire neocortex but at different layers than the RD. NA from the LC ends spontaneous firing of target neurons. The LC fires as a group and influences the entire brain simultaneously, that is, fast and bursty. Moreover, the LC output increases to new, aversive, or rewarding stimuli.

Signal propagation in LC neurons is comparatively slow, requiring 400 ms to reach the entire brain. During sleep, the LC outputs decrease and go to zero in REM sleep.

When the LC activity is high, the output of active nodes increases in all cortical modules and—by lateral interaction—depresses inactive nodes.

9

Philosophical Implications

NNs combines many disciplines. Previous chapters showed links among biology, psychology, physiology, control theory, signal processing, and nonlinear mathematics. This chapter considers philosophy.

Although sometimes controversial, philosophical issues are at the heart of many students' and researchers' interest in NNs, especially the nature of consciousness. This line of thought leads directly to some of the central philosophical questions debated since antiquity.

Because the chapter may be provocative, let me say outright that I wish to assert that NNs support a view of Aristotle regarding consciousness. NN theory also corrects a mistake made by philosophers about consciousness since the seventeenth century. The mistake started with Thomas Hobbes in England and René Descartes in France.

9.1 CONSCIOUSNESS

The subject of consciousness lies at the very basis of modern questions about the brain-mind of human beings. Indeed, human consciousness may be the last surviving mystery because people do not know how to think about it.

Without much reflection about it, most people suppose they are directly aware of the contents of their own minds, and they are when they feel pains, pleasures, and bodily strains. Such feelings, however, are different from quantities we call perceptions, memories, imaginations, dreams, and thoughts.

The words—pleasures, pains, feelings, perceptions, memories, imaginations, and thoughts—capture nearly all the conscious acts. To focus the discussion, following [2], consider the following question: When conscious, what are we conscious of?

The important word in the question is the preposition "of" that calls for an object. We customarily speak of the stream of consciousness, or flow of thought. Thus, an equivalent question is: What is the content of consciousness?

Historically, philosophers give two different answers to the question, not counting variations. As with technical subjects, some notation must be introduced.

John Locke introduced the term "idea." Idea in modern philosophy is applied in an omnicomprehensive fashion. Ideas refer to a variety of items including images, percepts, memories, thoughts, concepts, feelings, and sensations.

Returning to the question (When conscious, what are we conscious of?), Locke's answer is: When we are conscious all ideas are possible objects of our minds.

This answer, though reasonable at first glance, leads to several philosophical dead ends in the opinion of many. Consider the consequences. After long argument and discussion Locke's answer leads to absurdities, roughly as follows.

1. All ideas are the objects when conscious. (Locke)

2. Consciousness is a private experience.

3. Indeed, all ideas are private.

4. Each person is contained in their own private world.

5. So proving an external reality that agrees with other people's reality is impossible.

6. Thus, skepticism is complete regarding outside reality.

7. Alternatively, everything I am aware of is a figment of my own mind. (solipsism)

To avoid the absurd consequences of skepticism or solipsism, the argument is tried that ideas are representations, an argument, however, that leads to a contradiction. If people are aware of only ideas, reality can never be directly experienced. Indeed, their ideas cannot imitate reality because, say, a portrait can represent a person if and only if the portrait and the person can be compared. If the person is never seen, no claim of representation can be made.

Thus, Locke's answer about consciousness—and of many modern philosophers— leads to absurdity or contradiction.

Aristotle, and later Thomas Aquinas, gave another answer. To state this answer, define another term as follows.

Cognitive ideas are those ideas excluding feelings, emotions, and bodily sensations. That is, cognitive ideas are memories, concepts, and precepts. Cognitive ideas are the agent for apprehending the objects of consciousness. Thus, noncognitive ideas are feelings, emotions, and bodily sensations.

Returning to the question (When conscious, what are we conscious of?), Aristotle's answer is: When we are conscious, the objects of our minds are noncognitive ideas.

Interpreting this answer, while we can remember the feelings and sensations of past events, we are never aware of the memories or concepts by which we recall them.

A simple analogy is if memories are likened to a radio (cognitive ideas), we can hear messages (noncognitive ideas) produced by the radio, but we cannot know anything about the radio itself.

Again consider the consequences of this answer. After much argument and discussion, the answer leads to consequences that agree with experience and common sense.

1. When we are conscious, noncognitive ideas are the objects of our minds. (Aristotle)
2. Indeed, thoughts, experiences, and past events are the objects when conscious.
3. We are directly acquainted with the public existence of other people and objects.
4. Moreover, we can share noncognitive ideas, though we cannot share our cognitive ideas, because we are never conscious of them.

9.2 A NEURAL NETWORK INTERPRETATION

Readers of the previous chapters will immediately see a NN interpretation of the preceding notions.

Cognitive ideas are equivalent to—or are modeled by—the LTM traces in, say, ART-2. In NN terminology, Aristotle asserts people cannot be consciously aware of their own—or others'—LTM traces.

Once sensory experience—and other mechanisms—produce LTM traces, these patterns cannot be directly accessed.

The objects of consciousness—the flow of thoughts in our minds—are the STM patterns in NNs. Moreover, we are aware of only some of the STM patterns. Those STM patterns associated with, say, motor activity are usually unconscious.

9.3 FINAL REMARKS

Dennett [26] observed most brain researchers pretend that, for them, the brain is just another organ. Indeed, there is a reluctance to confront the "big issues," like consciousness.

Some researchers, feigning amnesia, pretend we do not have experiences we know full well we have. Others nitpick empirical details, such as some of Hubel and Wiesel's discoveries about vision.

Nonetheless, how the brain-mind works needs new ways of thinking. Neuroscience by itself is not enough, anymore than electronics is sufficient for understanding, say, virtual memory structures in modern computers.

NNs gives a viewpoint for developing and testing on machines new theories about phenomena in complex networks. Moreover, NNs helps organize coherent testable hypotheses.

The claim that a NN viewpoint is no possible explanation of the human brain-mind calls for showing what it has to leave out or cannot do. The claim that a NN model is incorrect in many details is conceded.

While NN modeling of higher processing is barely starting, nevertheless, its direction is clear: Philosophically speaking, NNs is a version of functionalism—that is, if you build the entire functional structure of the human brain, you would reproduce all the mental properties as well.

This introductory volume presents some of the necessary NN basics. Application of NNs for mimicking consciousness and higher-level mental processing may be the next major milestone.

SUGGESTED REFERENCES

M. ADLER, *Ten Philosophical Mistakes*. This book is a look at common errors in modern philosophical thought. The text summarizes the first chapter about consciousness. Later chapters discuss perceptual and conceptual thought, the source of word meanings, and the difference between opinion and knowledge.

G. EDELMAN, *Group Selection and Phasic Reentrant Signaling*: *A Theory of Higher Brain Function*. Most researchers believe all nervous systems obey similar principles in their mechanisms of signaling. At a functional level, however, confusion reigns. Indeed, until recently the neural structure for higher brain functions has been left to philosophical speculation and psychological testing. These efforts do not address the most challenging problem of neurobiology, namely the cellular mechanisms of higher brain functions, particularly consciousness. Edelman hypothesizes that consciousness results from stored patterns and current sensory input. Sensory and motor signals continually update consciousness. Sufficient conditions for conscious awareness include the quality of sensory inputs, something present theories of consciousness have not given. If a machine with these properties were built, it would report conscious states.

J. HAGELIN, *Is Consciousness the Unified Field? A Field Theorist's Perspective*. This paper, written by a theoretical physicist, proposes a unified field theory. The theory combines standard quantum mechanics with a field of "pure consciousness." Such a theory is consistent with all physical principles. It may account for experimentally observed field effects of consciousness. The paper is recommended as background.

D. DENNETT, *Consciousness Explained*. This recent work on consciousness has all the appearances of a typical nonscientific psychology work. Appearances are deceiving, however. The book is remarkably readable with a graceful, informal style that has fluency and notice of technical details. The central idea is that highly parallel processing, well known to the NN community, produces the phenomenon of consciousness. The book is highly recommended as background for this chapter, especially in comparison with Penrose's *The Emperor's New Mind*. Penrose suggests a revolution in physics is needed before consciousness is accessible to scientific investigation.

Glossary

Neuroanatomy Terms

Amygdala   A neural group in the dorsomedial temporal lobe bilaterally that enables learning in conjunction with the hippocampus.

Cerebellum   Part of the brain lying above brainstem that governs coordination of motor function and body orientation.

Cerebral cortex   The layer neurons covering the hemispheres on their external surfaces. The cortex supports many functions, including cognition. Called also the neocortex.

Corpus callosum   A large group of nerve fibers connecting the two cerebral hemispheres.

Dendrites   The branch-like structure of neurons that serves to sum impulses from other neurons.

Frontal lobe   The most forward part of the cerebral cortex enabling motor function and reasoning.

Interpreter   An area in the dominant hemisphere that seems to produce hypotheses and explanations about internal and external inputs.

Locus coeruleus   A group of about 1400 noradrenergic neurons in the brain stem that regulate attention and anxiety level.

Striatum   A group of neurons in the cerebral white matter, regulating motor programs and coordination. Inputs are from the substantia nigra, thalamus, and motor cortex. Outputs are to the hypothalamus, thalamus, and motor neural groups.

Synapse   The connection area between neurons through which signaling occurs.

Neuroscience Terms

Acetylcholine   An excitatory amine transmitter used throughout the nervous system. The transmitter is synthesized by the enzyme choline acetyltransferase from acetyl coenzyme A and choline and is metabolized by the enzyme acetylcholinesterase.

Amphetamines   A class of pharmacologic agents that release catecholamines from nerve terminals and inhibit the uptake and inactivation of amines. Amphetamine overdose may cause a paranoid psychosis.

Catalysis   Conversion of substances to products by an enzyme.

Catecholamine   A family of neurotransmitters defined chemically as 3,4-dihydroxy derivatives of phenylethylamines. Well-known members are dopamine, norepinephrine, and epinephrine.

Dopamine   A catecholamine neurontransmitter used by the substantia nigra neurons regulating motor function.

Enzyme   A molecule greatly increasing the rate of chemical reactions, without being permanently altered itself.

Epinephrine   A catecholamine neurontransmitter used by the adrenal medulla to regulate cardiovascular function in response to stress.

Gene   A unit of hereditary DNA molecule encoding a biological function.

Glia   Nonneural brain cells providing support and other functions.

Habituation   The decrease in synaptic efficiency from repeated exposure to a stimulus.

Ion channel   A large molecule or group of molecules inserted in the cell membrane forming a route for passage of particular charged molecules.

Long-term potentiation   Strengthening of synaptic efficiency by the simulataneous input signals to a neuron.

Serotonin   A neurotransmitter derived from dietary tryptophan that is localized in the raphe neurons of the brain stem and regulates sleep.

Philosophy Terms

Connectionism   A computational model of cognition where knowledge exists in the pattern and strengths of connections among elements, perhaps neural. Learning is the altering of the connections. Also termed *parallel distributed processing*.

Functionalism   The view that intelligence can be implemented by a variety of means, including computers.

Reductionism   The view that brain-mind functioning is explainable in terms of physical structure.

Psychology Terms

Conditioning, classical   The process of relating two stimuli, a conditioned and an unconditioned stimulus, resulting in a conditioned response.

Conditioning, instrumental   The process of relating the response and a reinforcing stimulus.

Bibliography

1. ACKLEY, D., HINTON, G., AND SEJOWSKI, T. 1985. A learning algorithm for Boltzmann Machines. *Cognitive Science* 9, 147–69.

2. ADLER, J. 1985. *Ten Philosophical Mistakes*. New York: Macmillan.

3. ADOMIAN, G., AND ADOMIAN, G. E. 1984. A global method for solution of complex systems. *Mathematical Modeling* 5, 251–63.

4. ANDREWS, R., AND STRINGER, C. 1989. *Human Evolution* (pp. 9–46). New York: Cambridge University Press.

5. BAILEY, C. H., AND GOURAS, P. 1981. The retina and phototransduction. In E. R. Kandel and J. H. Schwartz, eds. *Principles of Neural Science*, 2nd ed. (pp. 344–56). New York: Elsevier North-Holland.

6. BERLINSKI, D. 1976. *On Systems Analysis: An Essay Concerning the Limitations of Some Mathematical Methods in the Social, Political, and Biological Sciences*. Cambridge, MA: The MIT Press.

7. BICKEL, A., AND BICKEL, R. 1987. Tree structure rules in genetic algorithms. *Proceedings of the Second International Conference on Genetic Algorithms and Their Applications* (pp. 77–81). Palo Alto, CA: Morgan Kaufmann Publishers.

8. BLACK, I. 1991. *Information in the Brain*. Cambridge, MA: The MIT Press.

9. BLOOM, F. E., LAZERSON, A., AND HOFSTADTER, L. 1985. *Brain, Mind, and Behavior*. New York: W.H. Freeman.

10. BOSE, N. K., AND GARGA, A. K. 1992. Neural network design using Voronoi diagrams: Preliminaries. *Proceedings of the International Joint Conference on Neural Networks: Vol. 3* (pp. 127–38). Piscataway, NJ: IEEE Service Center.

11. BROGAN, W. L. 1974. *Modern Control Theory*. New York: Quantum Publishers, Inc.

12. BULLOCK, D., AND GROSSBERG, S. 1988. Neural dynamics of planned arm movements: Emergent invariants and speed-accuracy properties during trajectory formation. In S. Grossberg, ed. *Neural Networks and Natural Intelligence* (pp. 553–622). Cambridge, MA: The MIT Press.

13. CARPENTER, G. A. 1985. A neural theory of circadian rhythms: Split rhythms, after-effects and motivational interactions. *Journal of Theoretical Biology* 113, 163–223.

14. CARPENTER, G. A., AND GROSSBERG, S. 1987. A massively parallel architecture for a self-organizing neural pattern recognition machine. *Computer Vision, Graphics, and Image Processing* 37, 54–115.

15. CARPENTER, G. A., AND GROSSBERG, S. 1987. ART 2: Self-organization of stable category recognition codes for analog input patterns. *Applied Optics* 26, 4919–30.

16. CARPENTER, G. A., AND GROSSBERG, S. 1990. ART 3: Hierarchical search using chemical transmitters in self-organizing pattern recognition architectures. *Neural Networks* 3, 129–52.

17. CARPENTER, G. A., GROSSBERG, S., AND ROSEN, D. B. 1991. ART 2-A: An adaptive resonance algorithm for rapid category learning and recognition. *Neural Networks* 4, 493–503.

18. CASTI, J. L. 1977. *Dynamical Systems and Their Applications* (pp. 1–34). New York: Academic Press.

19. CELLIER, F. 1991. *Continuous System Modeling* (pp. 679–90). New York: Springer-Verlag.

20. SELBY, S. M. (Ed.) 1972. *CRC Standard Mathematical Tables*. 20th ed. Cleveland, OH: The Chemical Rubber Co.

21. CRICK, F. H. C., AND ASANUMA, C. 1988. Certain aspects of the anatomy and physiology of the cerebral cortex. In J. L. McClelland and D. E. Rumelhart, eds. *Parallel Distributed Processing: Vol. 2* (pp. 333–71). Cambridge, MA: The MIT Press.

22. DARNELL, J., LODISH, H., AND BALTIMORE, D. 1986. *Molecular Cell Biology* (pp. 625–28). New York: W.H. Freeman.

23. DARPA. 1988. *DARPA Neural Network Study—Final Report* (Technical Report 840). Lincoln, MA: MIT Lincoln Laboratory.

24. DEIMLING, K. 1985. *Nonlinear Functional Analysis* (pp. 186–216). New York: Springer-Verlag.

25. DE JONG, K. 1987. On using genetic algorithms to search program spaces. *Proceedings of the Second International Conference on Genetic Algorithms and Their Applications* (pp. 210–16). Palo Alto, CA: Morgan Kaufmann Publishers.

26. DENNETT, D. C. 1991. *Consciousness Explained*. Boston: Little, Brown.

27. The Diagram Group. 1987. *The Brain—A User's Manual*. New York: G. P. Putnam's Sons.

28. DUPRAW, E. J. 1968. *Cell and Molecular Biology* (pp. 266–70). New York: Academic Press.

29. EDELMAN, G. M., AND MOUNTCASTLE, V.B. 1982. *The Mindful Brain*. Cambridge, MA: The MIT Press.

30. FRISBY, J. P. 1980. *Seeing-Illusion, Brain and Mind*. New York: Oxford University Press.

31. GAUDIANO, P., AND GROSSBERG, S. 1991. Vector associative maps: Unsupervised real-time error-based learning and control of movement trajectories. *Neural Networks* 4, 147–83.

32. GOLDBERG, S. 1988. *Clinical Neuroanatomy Made Ridiculously Simple*. Miami, FL: MedMaster, Inc.

33. GROSSBERG, S., AND KUPERSTEIN, M. 1986. *Neural Dynamics of Adaptive Sensory-Motor Control: Ballistic Eye Movements*. New York: Elsevier Science Publishing Company, Inc.

34. GROSSBERG, S. 1982. *Studies of Mind and Brain*. Boston: D. Reidel Publishing Co.

35. GROSSBERG, S. 1988. Nonlinear neural networks: Principles, mechanisms, and architectures. *Neural Networks* 1, 17–61.

36. HAGELIN, J. S. 1987. Is consciousness the unified field: An introduction. *Modern Science and Vedic Science* 1(1), 29–87.

37. HARP, S. A., SAMARD, T., AND GUHA, A. 1989. Toward the genetic synthesis of neural networks. *Proceedings of the Third International Conference on Genetic Algorithms and Their Applications* (pp. 360–69). Palo Alto, CA: Morgan Kaufmann Publishers.

38. HARVEY, R. L., DICAPRIO, P. N., HEINEMANN, K. G., SILVERMAN, M. L., AND DUGAN, J. M. 1990. A neural architecture for potentially classifying cytology specimens by machines. *Proceedings of the Fourteenth Annual Symposium on Computer Applications in Medical Care* (pp. 539–43). Los Alamitos, CA: IEEE Computer Society Press.

39. HARVEY, R. L., AND HEINEMANN, K.G. 1991. A biological vision model for sensor fusion. *Proceedings of the 4th National Symposium on Sensor Fusion—Vol. 1* (pp. 119–29). Ann Arbor, MI: IRIA Center, ERIM.

40. HARVEY, R. L. 1991. Recent advances in neural networks for machine vision (Plenary paper). *Proceedings of the Third Biennial Acoustics, Speech, & Signal Processing Mini Conference* (pp. IV.1–IV.6). Weston, MA: IEEE Central New England Council.

41. HARVEY, R. L., DICAPRIO, P. N., AND HEINEMANN, K. G. 1991. A neural network architecture for general image recognition. *The Lincoln Laboratory Journal* 4, 189–207.

42. HARVEY, R. L., DICAPRIO, P. N., AND HEINEMANN, K. G. 1992. *A Neural Network Architecture for General Image Recognition* (Technical Report 955). Lincoln, MA: MIT Lincoln Laboratory.

43. HARVEY, R. M. 1993. Nursing diagnosis by computers: An application of neural networks. *Nursing Diagnosis* 4, 28–36.

44. HECHT-NIELSEN, R. 1990. *Neurocomputing* (p. 137). Reading, MA: Addison-Wesley.

45. HESTENES, D. 1987. How the brain works: The next great scientific revolution. In G. R. Smith and G. J. Erickson, eds. *Maximum Entropy and Bayesian Spectral Analysis and Estimation Problems* (pp. 173–205). Boston: D. Reidel Publishing Co.

46. HESTENES, D. 1992. A neural network theory of manic-depressive illness. In D. S. Levine and S. J. Leven, eds. *Motivation, Emotion, and Goal Direction in Neural Networks* (pp. 208–53). Hillsdale, NJ: Lawrence Erlbaum Associates.

47. HODGKIN, A. L., AND HUXLEY, A. F. 1952. A quantitative description of membrane current and its application to conduction and excitation in nerve. *J. Physiol.* 117, 500–544.

48. HOLLAND, J. 1975. *Adaptation in Natural and Artificial Systems.* Ann Arbor, MI: The University of Michigan Press.

49. HOPFIELD, J. J. 1982. Neural networks and physical systems with emergent collective computational abilities. *Proc. Natl. Acad. Sci. USA* 79, 2554–58.

50. HUANG, W. Y., AND LIPPMANN, R. P. 1987, June. *Comparisons between neural network and conventional classifiers.* Paper presented at the First International Neural Network Conference, San Diego, CA.

51. HUBEL, D. H. 1988. *Eye, Brain, and Vision.* New York: W.H. Freeman.

52. KANDEL, E. R., AND SCHWARTZ, J. H., eds. 1985. *Principles of Neural Science*, 2nd ed. New York: Elsevier North-Holland.

53. KENT, E. W. 1981. *The Brains of Men and Machines.* New York: McGraw-Hill.

54. KEYNES, R. D. 1979. Ion channels in the nerve-cell membrane. *Scientific American* 240(3), 126–35.

55. KOSKO, B. 1989. Unsupervised learning in noise. *Proceedings of the International Joint Conference on Neural Networks: Vol. I* (pp. 7–17). Piscataway, NJ: IEEE Service Center.

56. KUFFLER, S. W., NICHOLLS, J. G., AND MARTIN A. R. 1984. *From Neuron to Brain*, 2nd ed. Sunderland, MA: Sinauer Associates Inc. Publishers.

57. KUPERSTEIN, M. 1988. Neural model of adaptive hand-eye coordination for single postures. *Science* 239, 1308–11.

58. LI, H., AND KENDER, J. R., eds. 1988. Computer vision [Special Issue]. *Proceedings of the IEEE* 76(8).

59. LLOYD, J. M. 1975. *Thermal Imaging Systems*. New York: Plenum.

60. LIU, Z., GASKA, J. P., JACOBSON, L. D., AND POLLEN, D. A. 1992. Interneuronal interaction between members of quadrature phase and anti-phase pairs in the cat's visual cortex. *Vision Res.* 32, 1193–98.

61. LIPPMANN, R. P. 1987. An introduction to computing with neural nets. *IEEE ASSP Magazine* 4, 4–22.

62. LYNCH, G. 1986. *Synapses, Circuits, and the Beginning of Memory*. Cambridge, MA: The MIT Press.

63. MARR, D. 1982. *Vision*. San Francisco: W.H. Freeman.

64. MARTIN, K. A., AND PERRY, V. H. 1988. On seeing a butterfly: The physiology of vision. *Sci. Prog. Oxf.* 72, 259–80.

65. MAUNSELL, J. H. 1987. Physiological evidence for two visual subsystems. In L. Vaina, ed. *Matters of Intelligence* (pp. 59–88). Boston: D. Reidel Publishing Co.

66. MCCULLOCH, W., AND PITTS, W. 1943. A logical calculus of the ideas immanent in nervous activity. *Bulletin of Mathematical Biophysics* 5, 115–33.

67. MELZAK, A. A. 1976. *Mathematical Ideas, Modeling and Applications—Vol. II of Companion to Concrete Mathematics* (pp. 355–64). New York: John Wiley.

68. MILLER, G. F., TODD, P. M., AND HEGDE, S. U. 1989. Designing neural networks using genetic algorithms. *Proceedings of the Third International Conference on Genetic Algorithms* (pp. 379–84). San Mateo, CA: Morgan Kaufmann Publishers.

69. MILLER, R. F. 1988. Are single retinal neurons both excitatory and inhibitory? *Nature* 336, 517–8.

70. MILLER III, W. T., SUTTON, R. S., AND WERBOS, P. J., eds. 1990. *Neural Networks for Control*. Cambridge, MA: The MIT Press.

71. MINSKY, M., AND PAPERT, S. 1969. *Perceptrons*. Cambridge, MA: The MIT Press.

72. PASSINO, K. M., SARTORI, M. A., AND ANTSAKLIS, P. J. 1989. Neural computing for numeric-to-symbolic conversion in control systems. *IEEE Control Systems Magazine* 9(2), 44–52.

73. PENROSE, R. 1989. *The Emperor's New Mind*. New York: Oxford University Press.

74. POLLEN, D. A., GASKA, J. P., AND JACOBSON, L. D. 1989. Physiological constraints on models of visual cortical function. In R. M. J. Cotterill, ed. *Models of Brain Function* (pp. 115–35). New York: Cambridge University Press.

75. REES, A. R., AND STERNBERG, M. J. 1984. *From Cells to Atoms*. Boston: Blackwell Scientific Publications.

76. ROSE, D., AND DOBSON, V. G. 1985. *Models of the Visual Cortex*. New York: John Wiley.

77. ROSENFELD, A. 1987. Image analysis: problems, progress and prospects. In M.A. Fischler and O. Firschein, eds. *Readings in Computer Vision* (pp. 3–12). Los Altos, CA: Morgan Kaufmann Publishers.

78. ROSENFELD, A. 1988. Computer vision: Basic principles. *IEEE Proceedings* 76, 863–69.

79. RUMELHART, D., AND MCCLELLAND, J. 1986. *Parallel Distributed Processing*: *Vols. 1 and 2*. Cambridge, MA: The MIT Press.

80. SILVERMAN, M. L., DUGAN, J. M., HARVEY, R. L., DiCAPRIO, P. N., AND HEINEMANN, K. G. 1990, March. *A neural network as a potential means of reading cytology specimens*. Paper presented at the 79th annual meeting of The United States-Canadian Division of The International Academy of Pathology, Boston, MA.

81. SILVERMAN, M. L., DUGAN, J. M., HARVEY, R. L., DiCAPRIO, P. N., AND HEINEMANN, K. G. 1990, March. *Classification of individual cells by a neural network*: *A potential means of screening cytology specimens*. Poster presented at the 1990 Spring Meeting of the American Society of Clinical Pathologists, San Francisco, CA.

82. SHERIDAN, T. B., AND FERRELL, W. R. 1974. *Man-Machine Systems*. Cambridge, MA: The MIT Press.

83. VAN ESSEN, D. C., AND MAUNSELL, J. H. R. 1983. Hierarchical organization and functional streams in the visual cortex. *Trends Neurosci.* 6(9), 370–75.

84. WERBOS, P. J. 1974. Beyond regression: New tools for prediction and analysis in the behavioral sciences. Doctoral Dissertation, Applied Math, Harvard University.

85. WHITLEY, D., AND HANSON, T. 1989. Optimizing neural networks using faster, more accurate genetic search. *Proceedings of the Third International Conference on Genetic Algorithms* (pp. 391–96). San Mateo, CA: Morgan Kaufmann Publishers.

Figure Credits

The author gratefully acknowledges permission to reprint the following:

Figures 1.4, 2.1, and 2.7: From *Brain, Mind and Behavior* by Bloom, Lazerson, and Hofstadter. Copyright ©1985 by W.H. Freeman and Co. Reprinted by permission of W.H. Freeman and Co.

Figures 1.5, 1.6, and 2.2: From *The Brain—A User's Manual* by The Diagram Group. Copyright ©1982 and 1987 by Diagram Visual Information Limited. Reprinted by permission of Diagram Visual Information Limited.

Figures 2.4, 2.6, 2.9, 2.10, 5.1, and 8.1: From *From Neuron to Brain* (2nd ed.) by Kuffler, Nicholls, and Martin. Copyright ©1984 by Sinauer Associates, Inc.. Adapted (Figs. 2.4, 2.9) and reprinted (Figs. 2.6, 2.10, 5.1, 8.1) by permission of Sinauer Associates, Inc.

Figure 4.4: From "Nonlinear Neural Networks: Principles, Mechanisms, and Architectures" by Grossberg in *Neural Networks* **1**. Copyright ©1988 by S. Grossberg. Reprinted by permission of S. Grossberg.

Figures 4.12 and 4.13: From "ART 2: Self-Organization of Stable Category Recognition Codes for Analog Input Patterns" by Carpenter and Grossberg in *Applied Optics* **26**. Copyright ©1987 by G. A. Carpenter and S. Grossberg. Reprinted by permission of G. A. Carpenter.

Figure 5.2: From *Principles of Neural Science*, 2nd ed., by Kandel and Schwartz (eds.). Copyright ©1985 by Elsevier Science Publishing Co., Inc. Adapted, with permission, from the *Annual Review of Neuroscience* Vol. 2, ©1979 by Annual Reviews Inc., and by permission of Appleton & Lange and E.R. Kandel.

Index of Symbols

Index